T0251598

ACTION METHODS IN GROUP PSYCHOTHERAPY

ACTION METHODS IN GROUP PSYCHOTHERAPY

Practical Aspects

Daniel J. Tomasulo, Ph.D., T.E.P., CGP

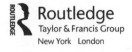

Routledge
Taylor & Francis Group
New York   London

First published 1998 by BRUNNER/ MAZEL Philadelphia and London

This edition published 2014 by Routledge
711 Third Avenue, New York, NY 10017
27 Church Road, Hove East Sussex BN3 2FA

Routledge is an imprint of the Taylor & Francis Group, an informa business

ACTION METHODS IN GROUP PSYCHOTHERAPY: Practical Aspects

Copyright © 1998 Taylor & Francis. All rights reserved. Except as permitted under the United States Copyright Act of 1976, no part of this publication may be reproduced or distributed in any form or by any means, or stored in a database or retrieval system, without prior written permission of the publisher.

A CIP catalog record for this book is available from the British Library.

Library of Congress Cataloging-in-Publication Data

Tomasulo, Daniel J.
    Action methods in group psychotherapy : practical aspects / Daniel
J. Tomasulo
    Includes bibliographic references and index.
    ISBN 1-56302-658-1. — ISBN 1-56203-659-X (pbk.)
BF637.C6T644 1998
158'.35—dc21   98-30865
                                                             CIP

ISBN: 1-56032-658-1 (cloth)
ISBN: 1-56032-659-X (paper)

TABLE OF CONTENTS

List of Figures

ACKNOWLEDGMENTS

First and foremost I wish to thank the people at Accelerated Development for inviting me to write this book. I am particularly thankful to Joe Hollis and Cindy Long for their patient and constructive manner in bringing this book to fruition.

Jacqueline Dubbs-Siroka, M.S.W., A.C.S.W., T.E.P., CGP, was my primary trainer in psychodrama. For the eight and a half years I studied with her, my admiration and awe of her ability and depth as a human being has given me inspiration. Beyond the technical information, Jackie provided the corrective model I needed in my life. She showed genuine compassion, admitted her faults, had integrity, was genuinely happy when something happened in my life that was good, and helped me through the pain when things went wrong. After all that time in training, I left feeling complete. What surprised me was that it was afterward, years later, that I felt the true power of Jackie's influence. My experience with her as my trainer served as a continual well-spring of growth for me—a touchstone that enabled me to draw from the reservoir of our encounters together to continue my own growth. It is both magical and profoundly human. Magical because I don't think I actually can describe exactly how it happened: How did watching and participating in a series of psychodramas that Jackie conducted over the years change me? Profoundly human because it gave me what we all need—someone who genuinely believes in us.

Bob Siroka, Ph.D., T.E.P., C.G.P., supervised me for both my New Jersey psychology license and my T.E.P. certification in psychodrama. The expanse of his knowledge, clarity of insight, and presence as a person were tremendously influential. Together Bob and Jackie became my psychodramatic parents. This is important to note because the therapeutic relationship that developed between us was the result of my being a member of Jackie's training group and Bob's supervision group, not the result of individual meetings. These group experiences offered me the opportunity to undergo the core revision of any group encounter, the corrective recapitulation of my primary family of origin.

Nancy Razza, Ph.D., CGP, is my wife, partner, and mother to our daughter, Devon. God apparently wanted me to have the opportunity to be loved and share my love with a woman who not only understands what makes me tick but has the same interests, goals, and desires I do in terms of our joint careers. I feel blessed to be part of this family and want to thank Nancy and Devon for giving me the time and encouragement I needed to write this book.

Along the way many friends and colleagues have inspired me. First is my long-time friend and colleague, Joel Morgovsky, who is doubly blessed as a psychologist and a photographer. He is credited with my photo at the back of this book. Anne Hurley, Al Pfadt, Perry Samowitz, Phil Levy, Joel Levy, Deb Wherlan, Jerry Weinstock, Ben Niven, and Rob Fletcher have been sources of encouragement and inspiration, and I greatly appreciate their encouragement, support, and influence in my development.

Finally, I would like to thank my trainees (particularly the Friday afternoon group) and group counseling students who, over the years, have motivated me to understand the magic that occurs when action methods are used in a group.

Daniel J. Tomasulo
May 1998

PREFACE

The author of any book on group psychotherapy has likely struggled with the question of what material to include and what to leave out. So it is with me. I have tried to offer a brief, and yet as thorough as possible, introduction to the world of action methods in group psychotherapy. However, I am aware that the needs of readers vary. As a reader, you may be pressed with the daunting task of starting a group, or if you are a seasoned professional, you may be faced with the challenge of adding action to your already existing group. To accommodate these diverse needs, I have included in the chapters on action methods and therapeutic factors exercises that should help you increase your awareness and develop your skill. For those who need a faster method of setting up and establishing a group, I have included in the final chapter, "Quick Start," a summary of information on how to begin and maintain a group, focusing on practical and functional material. The pressing need to deliver more services to more people with fewer dollars has put a spotlight on group psychotherapy. Action methods can maximize the psychotherapeutic experience in a brief time frame. My hope is that this book will serve as an accessible reference source for students and professionals. I invite your responses and reactions.

INVITATION TO AN ENCOUNTER

A meeting of the two: eye to eye, face to face
and when you are near I will tear your eyes out
and place them instead of mine,
and you will tear my eyes out
and will place them instead of yours,
and I will look at you with your eyes
and you will look at me with mine.

–Jacob Levy Moreno

As we consider group psychotherapy, many questions come to mind. How does group therapy work? How is group therapy different from individual therapy? From family therapy? Who runs groups? How do you learn to run a group? Are the laws governing individual psychotherapy the same as for group therapy? How many people should run a group? How many people should be in a group? Is group psychotherapy effective? Are short-term groups as good as long-term groups? How often should groups be run? Who joins a group? Can groups be harmful? Are there different theories of group work? Which theory is best? The list goes on and on.

1

This book will attempt to integrate what is known from the research about how groups work with what is known about the practical aspects of running effective groups. For the beginner, the basics will be identified, along with suggestions for avoiding pitfalls. For the seasoned professional, a host of techniques will be offered along with rationale for the use of these techniques.

Over the next decade, group psychotherapy will be used more and more in the treatment of psychological difficulties. Managed care, healthcare reform, and the Americans with Disabilities Act mandate the delivery of quality therapy for many people at a reasonable cost. Therefore, competent group psychotherapists will be needed.

Many kinds of groups have therapeutic value. Chapter 1 identifies different types of groups along with their respective goals and functions. The primary focus of this book, however, is on *applied* aspects of group work and on techniques that will enhance a broad range of group modalities. The main focus is on how to use action techniques to enhance the functioning of a group. The intent is to provide the novice in group psychotherapy with a usable handbook for working with therapeutic groups and to provide seasoned therapists with a variety of practical suggestions and a host of techniques that may be implemented into their practice.

The action methods I refer to also could be called "role-playing techniques." However, because everyone thinks they know what role-playing is, no one thinks they need guidelines for doing it. As a result, many clinicians stumble into using role-playing to amplify their work, and they then run into difficulty, use it ineffectively, or only realize a fraction of the impact they were hoping to achieve. My hope is that providing detailed information about how to use action techniques will allow clinicians greater success in using them.

Following Sam Keen's (1994) dictum that he does not trust any book that fails to provide some autobiographical comment from the author, I will share the specifics of my connection to group psychotherapy and psychodrama.

Upon graduating from Yeshiva University with a Ph.D. in Developmental Psychology, I sent a portion of my dissertation research to a conference held by the American Association for the Study of Mental Imagery. This organization had just been started by Joseph Shorr, and I was honored to be among the first to be chosen to present their studies. I was just beginning my teaching career and was preparing for the life of a college professor. The clinical or counseling "call" was not mine. Research and teaching were my desire.

At the conference, Jerome Singer, Ph.D., then director of the clinical psychology program at Yale University and a pioneer in the study of mental imagery (among other areas), took the time to say he liked the research I had done on the developmental aspects of imagery in children. He suggested I attend a clinical workshop being run at the conference by noted psychodramatist Shirley A. Barclay, M.S.W., T.E.P. He thought the action techniques of psychodrama would be of interest to me in my work on understanding the developmental aspects of imagery.

I would never be the same.

That four-hour workshop reawakened my psychological mindedness. I saw people who didn't know one another interact in ways that were profoundly moving, genuine, and dramatic. That workshop transformed me into a lifetime student of psychodrama. I wanted to learn how to do what Shirley had done.

When I returned to New Jersey from the conference in Los Angeles, I inquired about training in psychodrama. It was my good fortune that three of the perhaps most prominent psychodramatists working in the field lived in my county. In fact, one of these people, Nina Garcia, Ed.D., M.S.W., T.E.P., taught in the drama department of Brookdale Community College in Lincroft, New Jersey, where I just had begun to work. She was offering a course in psychodrama for the first time, and I enrolled.

Shortly after the course, I joined a psychodrama training group run by Jackie Siroka, M.S.W., A.C.S.W., T.E.P. The group was primarily for therapists who were interested in learning more about group psychotherapy and psychodrama. My initial intent was to join for a few months, learn everything I could about psychodrama and group therapy, and continue teaching. I ended up staying with the training group for eight and a half years. I later went through a retraining program to obtain a license as a counseling psychologist in the state of New Jersey and obtained certification as a psychodramatist along the way. Again I had been fortunate. Jackie Siroka's husband is Bob Siroka, Ph.D., T.E.P., a psychologist with a diplomat in counseling psychology and former president of the American Society for Group Psychotherapy and Psychodrama. He became my supervisor for group psychotherapy and for my psychology license in New Jersey. At about the same time, I was offered the opportunity to teach a group dynamics course at Brookdale Community College and a consulting job for the Monmouth Association for Retarded Citizens. I was drawn into the counseling field through psychodrama. Because of this, my way of thinking about human problems was through role theory, imagery, and action methods.

Over the years, I became more involved in consultations with various agencies. It became clear to me that the exceptionally powerful action techniques developed through psychodrama were not being used by many group therapists. It also became obvious that many of the hospitals and agencies needed to run groups for the patients they served but were not clinically prepared to do so. Somehow, offering group therapy was given a high priority, while clinical competency was either assumed or simply neglected.

My wife, Nancy Razza, Ph.D., CGP, is also a psychologist with training and supervision in psychodrama and group psychotherapy. We met about the time I went to the conference in Los Angeles, and our interests were very much the same. We shared a strong commitment to working with people with mental retardation. In the early 1980s, we began experimenting with providing group counseling to people with mild and moderate mental retardation. We realized that some people with a dual diagnosis of mental retardation and a psychiatric disability could benefit from a group with action/role-playing techniques as a central ingredient.

With the help of several people from the Young Adult Institute (Joel Levy, D.S.W., Phil Levy, Ph.D., Perry Samowitz, M.A., C.R.C., Ben Niven, and Jerry Weinstock, M.A.) as well as encouragement from researchers Al Pfadt, Ph.D. (1991) and Ellen Keller, Ph.D. (1995), I developed the Interactive-Behavioral Model for group counseling for people with mental retardation. This model uses modified action-oriented techniques and has enjoyed wide acceptance not only in the United States but in other countries as well. At the same time, my wife, Nancy Razza, began working with the Monmouth Association for Retarded Citizens and developed a training program using sociodrama and a modification of the Interactive-Behavioral Model to provide mentally retarded persons with sexual abuse avoidance training. Due to the success of these groups, I began offering training programs to help practitioners enhance their use of action methods with various populations in group settings. In organizing this, I was able to offer continuing education programs through the American Psychological Association at their national conferences. Several states, including Alaska, Georgia, Maryland, New Jersey, and Oregon, have had me train their therapists in action methods. In part, this book has evolved from these trainings. Many people have asked for a collection of my work on applying action methods and establishing inpatient and outpatient groups in different settings. This work is an attempt to respond to those requests as well as to offer to those not able to attend a training program the basics of using action techniques in group counseling.

There are other fine works on action techniques within the fields of psychodrama and sociodrama that I will refer to throughout the book. These are excellent resources for providing a deeper understanding of the theory and of how to target action methods for specific groups. This book differs from these others in that it is not focused on training psychodramatists. *Rather, the focus of this book is the direct application of action methods in a wide variety of contexts in many forms of group work.* This book presents the indications and contraindications of various action procedures. It gives techniques that, when used in the proper context and with good supervision, will enhance your clinical group skills.

The book is divided into 10 chapters and contains 2 appendices.

Chapter 1 offers a brief overview of practical suggestions for beginning a group and theoretical issues important to groups.

Chapter 2 gives a detailed description of the basics, that is, four of the most essential action methods available to a group leader: the double, the empty chair, use of the auxiliary, and role reversal.

Chapter 3 provides a description of therapeutic factors that have been determined to be powerful indicators of a group's therapeutic viability.

Chapter 4 presents a complete transcript and analysis of a training group in which basic techniques were employed. This transcript includes processing notes and a description of the methods used and why.

Chapter 5 focuses on understanding the mechanics of group process when action techniques are used.

Chapter 6 returns to the transcript and processing of the training group.

Chapter 7 provides detailed information on the use of various techniques with groups larger than 20 people.

Chapter 8 applies action techniques to severely disabled people. It is designed to demonstrate the usefulness of action methods with diverse populations.

Chapter 9 provides a verbatim transcript of a group using the Interactive-Behavioral Therapy (IBT) format along with process and commentary.

Chapter 10 presents "Quick Start," a brief summary of how to begin and maintain a group.

Appendix A is a glossary. Selected terms throughout the book are highlighted and defined.

Appendix B, "Resources," includes books, journals, training programs, and certification programs available internationally.

PRACTICAL SUGGESTIONS FOR BEGINNING A GROUP

TYPES OF GROUPS

Outpatient or Inpatient

Before detailing how to start a group, we should consider the distinctions among different types of groups. Perhaps the broadest distinction is between outpatient and inpatient groups. Outpatient groups operate in private practice or agency-affiliated settings such as hospitals, schools, and human service agencies. Inpatient groups operate in restricted areas such as hospitals or residential facilities and usually serve those with chronic or acute care needs.

Private Practice or Agency-Affiliated Groups

Another distinction is between private practice and agency-affiliated groups. Although many of the same principles will apply to running a group in your private practice or for an agency (by "agency" it is meant any hospital, human service facility, school, community program, etc.), there are some very important differences. When running a group for an agency, you may have little

9

say in your readiness or ability to run a group, patient selection, schedule, time, patient removal, supervision, or ongoing training. Often people with little or no experience are asked to run a group, and they are given this responsibility by their agency with little help in the way of guidelines. The following situations are all too familiar.

> **Case of Patricia.** One month on the job, she complained that the large number of adolescents in the partial hospitalization program were not being assigned to treatment programs properly. She suggested that therapy groups be organized as part of the program. Her supervisors agreed that was a good idea and directed her to begin two therapy groups for the adolescents in the program. Patricia had never taken a single course in group therapy and just had begun her first semester in graduate school. Being thrown into the role of facilitator without training doomed her and the group to failure.

> **Case of Peter.** Peter was a group psychotherapist who was being supervised by a psychiatrist. He became aware that the supervisions were less than adequate and asked the psychiatrist how much experience he had had in running groups. The psychiatrist revealed that 20 years earlier he had run groups during a 10-week rotation on an inpatient unit. He said he intensely disliked the experience and vowed never to run a group again. While he was a very competent psychiatrist, known for giving valuable consultations, his group skills were inadequate, to say the least. Peter and his supervisor jointly agreed to bring in outside consultation on a monthly basis.

If you are asked to run a group within an agency, the eight guidelines offered in Figure 1.1. will increase your group's chances for success.

As a private practitioner, you have more options about the population with whom you work and the parameters surrounding your group work.

Figure 1.1. Guidelines for beginning a group in an agency.

1. Talk to the administration before you begin the group. Explain what you will need in terms of autonomy (letting people into and out of the group) and support (co-facilitation, supervision, transportation problems of members, emergency back-up, and absenteeism). Try to anticipate problems and ask about procedures ahead of time. Beginning with an open dialogue is the best way to head off trouble.

2. Create a group that you will feel comfortable handling. Select people that you feel good about and those with whom you feel you might have rapport. If you do not know the people, try to get to know those you are considering for the group prior to their admission. If you are co-facilitating, choose a person with whom you enjoy working.

3. Keep the number of people in the group small—six or seven to begin with.

4. If at all possible, work with a co-facilitator. Even if your co-facilitator is a silent partner, another pair of eyes and ears to help you process the group afterward will be helpful.

5. Ask for (demand!) supervision at least weekly from your clinical supervisor. Keep your supervisor informed of your progress or lack of it in the group. Competent supervision is essential for the functioning of a viable group.

6. Process the group after each session. If you are working with a co-facilitator, review the dynamics of the group together. If possible, obtain the proper releases and make videotapes of as many group sessions as you can. A videotape enhances the supervision and learning that can come from your work. It also provides an opportunity to show concrete examples of patient progress over time. This will help elevate your awareness and help you prepare for the next session. An audiotape of the session (with proper release forms) is also helpful; however, a video reveals more subtleties of the group process. From time to time, a transcript of the session may yield insights into dynamics that may have been overlooked during the session.

Continued

Figure 1.1. Guidelines for beginning a group in an agency (*Continued*)

---

7.   Request that some of your training money in the agency be used to send you to a conference or workshop on group therapy. There is probably no better way to learn than to talk with people with more or different experience than yours.

8.   Announce the beginning of your group to others in your facility. Whenever you institute a change in an agency, it is best to let others know of your intentions. Often such an announcement can head off difficulties later on.

Homogeneous or Heterogeneous

Another distinction is between homogeneous and heterogeneous groups. In *homogeneous* groups, all members of the group have similar problems. In *heterogeneous* groups, members have different problems and are in different life stages. An example of a homogeneous group is a group for recently divorced women or a group of recovering alcoholics. The advantage of homogeneous groups is that the support members can lend to one another. A homogeneous group is likely to develop cohesion (see Chapter 3, Therapeutic Factors) sooner than a heterogeneous group, because people with similar problems are likely to understand and empathize with each other more readily. A heterogeneous group can add diversity and depth to the dynamics of the group because no one common factor is universal to all members.

Once you have determined the type and focus of the group you can accept or decline membership based on these criteria. The more restrictive the criteria the more homogeneous your group. The more global your theme the greater the heterogeneity. A group for adults from a dysfunctional family of origin is going to be more diverse than a group of adolescent substance abusers. Groups for only women or only men add a dimension of trust and safety to the process. However, such restrictions limit the rich interactions that come from mixing both sexes. Choosing to run a homogeneous rather than heterogeneous group does not guarantee ease or success.

Once you have decided on the type of your group, you are ready to choose group members. Listed below is a sample of specialty groups randomly selected from recent journal articles. The list is by no means exhaustive. There could be as many types of groups as there are classifications of individuals with needs.

- Adults from dysfunctional families
- Grieving adults
- Divorced adults
- Adolescents
- Women's issues
- Men's issues
- Substance abuse
- Codependents
- Gay issues
- HIV groups
- Pregnant teens
- Eating disorders
- Mentally retarded young adults
- Multiproblem young adults
- Psychiatric outpatients

Open, Closed, or Psychoeducational

Other types of groups are open, closed, and psychoeducational. In an *open group*, you determine the size of the group and as members "graduate" or drop out, you replace them. A *closed group* is not open to new members and usually runs for a set period of time. A *psychoeducational group* is designed primarily to provide information to its members. This type of group works well for people with alcoholism early in their recovery.

Each of these formats has pros and cons. An open group has the advantage of mimicking life. People move in and out of the group as a microcosm of the way life really is. Some people move through it successfully, and their success instills hope in the membership. Others drop out without a trace—never to be heard from again. In the best of all worlds, you do not want this to happen. But the universe being what it is, it may. Then it becomes "grist for the mill," and the membership deals with the feelings of loss. On the other hand, when people leave, new people come into the group and provide new views, new connections, and new chemistry—all of which add to the richness of the group's life.

A closed group provides a measure of safety and security not available to an open group. The members know one another and know that there is no opportunity for others to attend the group meetings. This usually heightens the cohesion of the group and emphasizes the confidentiality among the members.

Many people use psychoeducational groups as a pre-group experience.

A hospital set up a 10-week psychoeducational program for people on their waiting list for group therapy. This provided a solution to several problems they faced:

1. A 28% increase in the number of referrals had occurred in the past six months.

2. At the same time, a 10% reduction had occurred in the staff.

3. People on the waiting list were getting lost after months of not being contacted.

4. Interns wanted the experience of working with people in a group setting.

5. A need existed to determine which people would be viable candidates for group counseling.

During this 10-week program of one and a half hour sessions, such topics as "Understanding Dysfunctional Families" and "Dealing with Addiction" were covered. The interns developed the topics and provided a discussion to follow. By offering a psychoeducational group, this hospital was better able to meet the needs of the community. The waiting list was reduced, and group facilitators had the opportunity to evaluate the group members and direct them toward the most appropriate follow-up treatment.

As a group practitioner, the problems you are trying to solve may be quite different. However, providing a short-term psychoeducational format may be an effective way to market your services while providing an educational opportunity for your community.

PREPARATION

Before beginning any group, first obtain, if you don't already have it, sufficient training and credentials to begin the kind of group you wish to start. Academic preparation may include one undergraduate and one graduate course (finding more than one course in any master's level academic program is rare) in a degree program in human services, psychology, social work, nursing, rehabilitation, or a related counseling field.

Second, you may wish to join a self-study or other *training group* of some sort. Generally speaking, very little academic preparation for running groups is offered. Some clinical counseling programs in psychology have a three-credit course devoted to group *and* family therapy! Do not expect to learn everything you need to know from these courses. Think of them as giving you a "license to learn," and then look outside the universities for membership in a training group. Such membership is highly valuable and will provide you with empathy for members in your group. A list of professional organizations that provide training in group psychotherapy appears in Appendix B. In recent years, the idea of certification in group psychotherapy has caught on, and the credential *CGP (Certified Group Psychotherapist)* now is being awarded to those meeting criteria of training and supervision.

Third, obtain a good group psychotherapy supervisor, someone with significantly more group experience than you. This person should have familiarity with the population you are planning to serve. It is often the case that supervisors of group psychotherapy have little background in group dynamics. If you are working for an agency that does not provide adequate supervision, ask about the possibility of bringing in a consultant. If you have these three ingredients—academic preparation, ongoing personal group experience, and good supervision—your efforts are likely to be effective.

Bernard and Mackenzie (1994) offered an organized presentation in which competence in patient selection may be gained. Their guidelines for facilitators seeking necessary training include the following:

1. Formal training

   Designated supervisor

   Criteria of competence identified

   Certificate of competence awarded

   A. Apprenticeship model

       Clinical setting with a clinical population

       Supervisor closely monitors clinical work and leads discussion of didactic material

   B. Continuing education model

       Professional workshops and conferences with nonclinical population

       Supervisor facilitates didactic discussion and leads experiential process groups

2. Informal training

   Local settings with clinical population

   Peer supervision through tapes, clinical notes, or in vivo

   Expert consultant for in services

   Record keeping for continual appraisal of procedures (p. 28)

My final suggestion has to do with remembering the larger group of which we are all a part. Purchase malpractice insurance before you begin. In our litigious society, even if you have done everything right with the people you serve, you may find yourself paying for a lawyer. Find insurance through your professional organizations or be sure your facility has made provisions for you to be insured. While group psychotherapy remains one of the lowest insurance risks to date, you should protect yourself with coverage. Costs vary depending on your credentials and professional associations.

SAFETY AMONG MEMBERS

The trust and safety people feel in the group will be one of the most important features of their group experience. Very little can be accomplished if group members do not have at least a minimal sense of trust and safety with one another and with the facilitator. Some of the action techniques identified throughout this book can be used to establish such a sense of safety among group members.

Case of Janet. This is an example of a group without safety. As a young woman early in her own therapeutic work for recovery from an incest memory, and with essentially no credentials at all, Janet started a "support group" which she facilitated and for which she charged members of the group—women who were sexual abuse victims. In no time, this group became unsafe and harmful to its participants. Janet, in leading the group, invited too much self-disclosure too soon from her members. The volume, intensity, and depth of the material shared was too much for an unskilled facilitator to handle. Ultimately, the women in the group had to seek therapy to recover from the "support group." When asked, Janet said that she had thought she would have no trouble running the group because everybody in it had the same background. She wrongly assumed that a common bond was a sufficient condition for success.

FREQUENCY AND LENGTH

Frequency and length of meeting time are two other considerations in planning a group. Outpatient private group therapy meetings are most often held weekly, with an average time of one and a half to two hours. There are no hard and fast rules about frequency or length. Some groups meet every other week for two and a half hours; others meet once a week for an hour. In the addiction field, meetings often are held twice a week or more. An important factor to consider when determining the frequency and length of your group meetings is your personal rhythm.

> **Case of Martha.** Martha, a psychologist, ran her women's group weekly for an hour and a half. After several months, it became clear to her that she needed more time for the group to function effectively. She felt she could not get the work done with the time originally planned. She opened this issue up to the group, and there was a general agreement that adding an extra half hour to the weekly sessions was worth trying. The change in the structure of the group was an empowering event for its members as well as for Martha. By choosing to make a change and then acting on it, the group was able to define the mechanics that worked for them.

SELECTING MEMBERS

Choosing the members for your group involves many considerations. If you are a private practitioner looking to put together a group of 10 members, you should gather about 25 people who are interested in joining a group. A natural attrition takes place along the route to becoming a group member. Hospitals, schools, and residential facilities may not have as much attrition because their populations are drawn from a more readily accessible group. Primary considerations in forming either a homogeneous or a heterogeneous group include availability of the clients at the hours and location where the group is held, readiness to be a member, client goals, and client deviance.

Availability

People living more than an hour away from the group or whose jobs would cause regular disruptions will have difficulty in being assimilated into groups. Scheduling conflicts with other meetings, transportation problems, and prior commitments are all potential indicators of problems. These issues should be resolved before admission is allowed.

Readiness

The potential members' interest in joining a group is often a measure of their psychological readiness. Determine the motivation of the people who are seeking to enter the group. What have they heard about group therapy? About you? What are their fears? Can they make a reasonable commitment to the group for a pre-scribed number of sessions? (It is reasonable to ask for 3 to 10 sessions as a commitment.) Consider the backgrounds of those preparing to join the group. If most have had extensive individual treatment or have been in group therapy before, you may want to be sure that all who enter the group have some degree of psychological mindfulness. On the other hand, if new members are all relatively new to the group experience, each can start on an equal footing. Answers to such questions will enable you to determine how people will fit into your newly forming group.

Woods and Melnick (1979) put forth guidelines as selection criteria for group members (Figure 1.2). Although it has been several years since these criteria have been identified, they still reflect the core elements of a candidate's readiness criteria. A slightly more recent perspective (Poeys, 1985) adds to those guidelines listed in Figure 1.2. Poeys' list is shown in Figure 1.3.

Goals

Each member should have identifiable goals that they wish to tackle in the group. These goals can, of course, change, and they may be somewhat nebulous (e.g., I want to learn why I have problems with relationships), but they will serve as a focus. Those

---

- Minimum level of interpersonal skill

- Motivation for treatment

- Positive expectations of gain from therapy

- Current psychological discomfort

- An interpersonal problem

- Commitment to changing interpersonal behavior

- Susceptibility to the group influence (moderate approval dependency)

- Willingness to be of help to others.

Source: Woods & Melnick, 1979, p. 162

Figure 1.2. Selection criteria for group members.

wishing to join a group but are uncertain of their reasons should spend at least a few individual session with the facilitator to help clarify their direction. Those who are joining solely because they were told to by someone else (a therapist, a spouse, etc.) are usually the most difficult to assimilate into the group process. It is strongly recommended that you meet with these people individually to see if they can identify reasons of their own for wanting to join your group. If they cannot, another course of action can be explored.

Deviance

Each group is like a mini-culture. You must take care not to put someone in a group who is too different from the norm for that group, otherwise they will become alienated from others in the group.

> **Case of Anna.** A generally high-functioning professional woman wished to join a group. She was an ideal candidate but could not attend on the evening of the most appropriate group. She was, however, avail-

able on an evening in which a group with a number of severely traumatized members had an opening. Although the facilitator told her that she would not really fit into that group, she insisted, and the facilitator agreed against his better judgment. By the second meeting it became clear that due to her healthier level of functioning, she was the most deviant person in the group. This was predictable and preventable. Had the facilitator stuck with his original sense of her needs, he would have placed her in a different group with a colleague or waited until she was available on the night with the more appropriate group.

Anna had had antagonistic relationships with almost every member of her family. In addition, she had antagonistic relationships at work, and all of her personal relationships with men were disappointing and unfulfilling. She wanted to get into a group but was unaware that a group would be not only a source of support but also a challenging mirror of her development within her family of origin. She was not aware of the rich dynamics that take place in the group. Prior to her entrance into the group, the fact that her antagonistic relationships were likely to reemerge in the group set-

---

- Ability to verbalize a focal complaint
- Significant level of psychological mindedness
- Urge to grow and explore
- Desire to enter a (short-term) group
- Realistic expectations of the group
- Basic ability to relate to and be influenced by others

Source: Poeys, 1985, in Bernard & Mackenzie, 1994, p. 20

Figure 1.3. Additional selection criteria for group members.

ting was discussed. Indeed, she was told that it was likely for this to happen if she was to successfully move through the group process. She had spent almost five years in an all-woman support group. Despite efforts to explain that a psychodynamic group was likely to have deeper inter-active properties than a homogeneous support group, she wanted to join. She felt she would not experience the kind of antagonism she knew in other quarters; how-ever, by her fifth meeting, she felt alienated and frus-trated by the experience. She had become deeply em-broiled in a series of antagonistic arguments with mem-bers. Despite her obvious intelligence, her ability to grasp emotional insight into these matters was nonexistent. She could not see how she played a role in the antagonistic attitude of the members. She was the least psychologi-cally minded individual in the group with regard to in-sight into her own behavior. On several occasions she was given very loving yet honest feedback about her behavior, but her personality was such that she could not assimilate this information and as a result she left the group.

Case of Michael. An exceptionally bright man with two Ph.D.s, one in physics and one in literature, was seeking membership in a group. Although Michael's depressive manner was obvious, the facilitator was dis-tracted from Michael's deeper emotional difficulties be-cause of his intelligence. He was placed in a high func-tioning group of people who related through strong in-teractions and constructive confrontation with each other. Within three meetings it was clear that although he was exceptionally bright, Michael's emotional need greatly exceeded what the group was willing to offer. He was removed by the facilitator and placed in a group more suited to his emotional state.

To date, no foolproof method has been identified for matching up the right person to the right group. Giving potential members an honest appraisal of likely difficulties and benefits is essential prior to their entering the group. The previously listed guidelines (Figures 1.2 and 1.3) offer some help in this selection process.

SIZE OF THE GROUP

The appropriate size for the group is, to some degree, dependent upon the skill level of the facilitator. However, some basic guidelines may be helpful. Ten people is a reasonable number to include in a group. The ideal number is about eight, with a low threshold of six. Usually two or three people are absent from any session. If you have a cofacilitator, you may be able to manage more people in the group, but it is best to have a smaller number when starting out. In the first group you run, you will be developing your skills as helping the members of the group. It is best to have six well-chosen, highly motivated people who are ready for a group experience. Although not a hard and fast rule, the greater the psychiatric disability of the membership, the smaller the group should be.

PHYSICAL SETTING

The room you use should have privacy and adequate seating for three more people than you plan to have in a circle. There should be no chairs or tables in front of anyone in the group. This will block their work, particularly if you plan to use action techniques. The chairs should be durable, firm, yet not overly comfortable. Too much comfort inhibits group work. Too little distracts. Close proximity of a restroom and water cooler will provide the group with adequate psychical comfort for the duration of the group. Safety is another important consideration. Usually your groups will be held in the evening, when regular office hours for many of your building occupants will be over. Take care that proper lighting of the parking lot and building hallways is provided during the time your group meets. Some office buildings have automatic timers for their air conditioning, heating, lighting, and security systems. Be sure these services are available for you when your groups are planning to run. The availability of a phone (for emergencies) and an awareness of the electrical panel (to reset circuit breakers) are also good ideas. If you are holding the group in your home, it should be in a separate area from the rest of the house to maintain healthy boundaries. You also should check limits of your home insurance. While these concerns may seem trivial to the reader, each has caused a disruption in my running a group at one time or another.

Finally, note the parking restrictions that may be placed on your facility. One practitioner was about to purchase an exceptional office building in a good part of town but backed out of the deal when he learned that the town only permitted six cars to be parked in the lot at any one time (even though the lot could accommodate twice that number). The practitioner was primarily a group psychotherapist and needed more than the six spaces allotted. Some locations may give you a variance for this, but check with an attorney before going through with your transaction.

EXECUTIVE FUNCTIONS

Decisions about your group are entirely up to you when you are operating as a private practitioner. Below are some of the common decisions for which a private practitioner is responsible:

- Who gets into the group
- Who must leave
- What the procedures are for terminating membership in the group
- What the rules of the group are
- How long the group will run
- What the fees are
- What time the group will start
- What time the group will end
- How (and if) new members will join the group

- What the purpose of the group is

- How confidentiality will be handled

- How intragroup relationships are to be handled

- Advanced schedule of holidays and canceled meetings

- Telephone list (if appropriate)

Each practitioner must decide on each of these factors as a way of preparing for the group. How you will screen members for inclusion right through to the termination process are all issues that must be decided upon prior to beginning. Over time, each group becomes like a separate culture. It has its own internal rules and rhythms that are evidenced by the interaction among the members. The rules and decisions you establish in the beginning help determine the evolution of that culture.

For example, if you do not address the issue of whether or not members can have outside relationships with one another, you run the risk of having to establish a rule after something happens that you did not want to happen. If you do allow members to connect with others outside of the group, it will be important that you inform them that all member-to-member contact outside of group should be reported back to the group so as not to create "in group" and "out group" experiences. Failure to stipulate this rule in the beginning (and each time a new member joins) is an error. If you do not want members interacting with each other outside of group (as might be the case in some psychoanalytic groups, for example), you should identify this rule and the ramifications for breaking it.

CONFIDENTIALITY ISSUES

One of the most important aspects of group functioning is *confidentiality*. Confidentiality is a topic that must be raised repeatedly in an ongoing group. This is particularly true when it is an open group and a new member joins. Provisions for confidentiality are different depending on the type of group you are running.

They may also be different with special populations and with children. For adult outpatient, private practice groups, the confidentiality issue should be addressed in the opening moments of the first group with a statement that covers six basic features:

1. In most instances, members in the group have the right to decide what to say and if to say anything. While some groups might require members to speak, these groups usually are outside the domain of the private practice facilitator. Such highly structured groups are much more likely to be used in inpatient group psychotherapy. (See Yalom, 1983, for a complete review of inpatient group process.) The work in the group is for people to say their thoughts and feelings and why they are having them. Toward this end, people will be encouraged to speak, but the decision remains with each person.

2. In order for the group to function properly, people must maintain the confidential needs of those in the group. What a person reveals in a group must not be discussed outside of the group.

3. If a breech of confidentiality does occur, it must be brought to the facilitator's attention as soon as possible.

4. The facilitator does not have control over members in the group, so each person is responsible for maintaining the confidentiality of the group. Members must make and stick to this commitment as part of their membership in the group.

5. Procedures for dealing with these issues and penalties for breaking confidentiality exist. For example, speaking up about the issue in group might be a procedure and expulsion from the group might be a penalty.

6. Members need to know that it is okay and, in fact, necessary for them to talk about what went on in the group with certain significant others. However, in continuing

their work outside of the group, they must comply with three essential rules:

a. Preserve the anonymity of the group members when they refer to them.

b. Mask the details of what was revealed by making them general rather than specific.

c. Share their own reactions to what was revealed, not what was actually revealed.

Case of Mary and John.   Mary is talking in the group about the kind of abuse she received from her mother. Mary offers great detail about this abuse and is distraught while telling it. If John hears this and is reminded of the abuses he experienced from his father, but does not share this with the group, he may feel the need to talk about it with his sponsor, therapist, or wife. If he does talk to *anyone* about it, he should focus on what came up for him. If need be, he could begin with a very general statement like "Someone in group was talking about the abuse she received as a child and it made me think of my abuse" as a way of introducing his information. In this way the anonymity of the group member is kept intact while John is able to continue his work outside of group.

In such a way, individual members continue the work begun in the group, while confidentiality is maintained.

FINANCIAL FACTORS

Financial issues are more often a problem if you are in private practice. Generally speaking it is a good idea to have one standing fee for all your group sessions. A group session of one and a half to two hours is usually priced at about half of the going individual rate. The fees you set for a group session should be consistent for all group members, with the understanding that if there is difficulty with the fee you would discuss it with each person individually. It is reasonable to expect that you may have to arrange a modification of your fee with some members. Keep in mind that any arrangement that you make with a group member is likely to be public. It is not reasonable or, for that matter, therapeutic, to make a financial arrangement with someone and expect them to keep it a secret. While it is certainly not the facilitator's role to announce the different financial arrangements, it is very likely that they will be revealed by the members themselves. The facilitator must be prepared to explain the reason for the differences in the fees.

> **Case of Harry.** Harry, a group member who had been in the group for about a year, told the group that he had decided to quit because of financial reasons. He had made significant progress in the group, and it was evident that he most needed to continue the group work during the time he was least able to afford it. He was told during group (since he brought it up) that if he wanted to talk with the facilitator afterward, it could be determined if an alternate arrangement could be agreed upon. The facilitator then took that opportunity to explain that this was something he would be willing to extend to all group members if the need arose. The facilitator also took the opportunity to explain two options that had been arranged with other people from different groups. One was a deferred payment option, whereby a partial payment was made by the group member and a deferment of the balance was made until the member was back on her feet. The other was reduced fees for a period of time with the understanding that once the individual was able to pay the usual rate he/she would resume payments at that rate.

Some facilitators have used creative means for establishing groups. One such method is to form a free, short-term (10-week) group with people who are in individual therapy with you. This enables you to get the group off and running. During the 10 weeks, continue to recruit additional members. This should ensure enough members continue with the group in the same weekly time slot once the 10 weeks are done. Another idea is that once you have a group going, offer three free group sessions to any individual you feel would add a good mix to the group.

One method is to charge a flat monthly fee for group. Thus, members are charged for the groups whether or not they show up. Another method is to charge on a per session basis. While the first way is convenient for bookkeeping and was designed to compel members to deal with their resistance, in the long run it may prove to be more cumbersome to manage. Most managed care programs need specific dates for services with a fee for each service offered. In this case, the "flat rate" still needs to be broken down into a weekly rate. Also, few insurance carriers and fewer managed care companies will reimburse for missed sessions.

Managed Care

Broadly speaking, "managed care" is neither. There are a wide variety of managed care programs. Nearly without exception they tend to be disorganized, inefficient, and concerned almost exclusively with financial factors. (The exceptions to date have been those managed care facilities operated by the professionals providing the service.) This is likely due to the infancy of managed care in mental health. Managed care isn't strictly oxymoronic, and it is a reality that you will likely have to face when developing an outpatient practice. If you pick up almost any professional newsletter you will see that the topic of managed care is well represented. Many psychotherapists have left managed care programs for a variety of reasons. Some reasons were that the programs were doing something unethical or illegal. Other reasons were strictly financial.

Case of Dena. One managed care program cut their fee structure almost 60% with no warning or indication they were going to do so. Dena, the therapist, found out about it only when she submitted her bill. This was months after the patient had been coming. When she asked to see a copy of the fee schedule, she was told it was privileged and confidential information and that she couldn't get it!

We've all heard many unfavorable stories from providers about managed care. Generally, mental health providers feel they are lucky if they get paid for their services at all. The one bright spot in the picture is that group psychotherapy seems to have become the darling of managed care. A number of the top managed care programs have endorsed the Certified Group Psychotherapist (CGP) credential. Also, it appears that the fee paid for group psychotherapy is closer to market value than the cost reimbursement of individual care.

Here are some practical guidelines for involvement with managed care:

- Talk to other providers about which managed care organizations have been most cooperative. Remember that providers with credentials different from yours may have different pay schedules and different requirements. Be sure the information you get is from someone with credentials similar to yours.

- Talk directly with provider services for the managed care company you wish to join. Have them send you a provider's application packet and rate schedule.

- Review the package *completely* once you have received it. Look for information about the reports you have to file (often called *Outpatient Treatment Reports [OTRs]*) and how often they must be filed. Of particular importance is to note *when* the report must be filed.

One managed care provider will only certify six sessions of group psychotherapy at a time yet requires a four-week lead time before sessions can be authorized. An example of the schedule for someone needing longer than six sessions in the group for this particular managed care company would be as follows:

a. *Initial individual evaluation session*: Send in the OTR and request authorization for six sessions of group psychotherapy. The initial evaluation session must be identified specifically by something called a CPT (Current Procedural Terminology) procedure code # 90801. Writing on the form that this is an initial evaluation will not suffice. The CPT code number tells the managed care company what you are doing and for how long you are doing it. The 90801 code is for an individual session for a duration of up to an hour.

b. *You then must wait for approval before the person can begin group work:* If you start the person in group prior to authorization, you run the risk of not having the fee for the session covered, and you may not be able to charge the client for this session due to your contract with the managed care provider.

c. *Second group session:* You now must send the OTR into managed care requesting additional sessions. This is necessary to continue past the sixth session.

d. *You then must wait for approval before the person can continue beyond the sixth session:* If you do not do so, you run the risk of not having the fee beyond the sixth session covered. As before, you most likely will not be able to charge the client for these sessions due to your contract with managed care. Once approved you may continue beyond the sixth session.

e. *Eighth group session:* You must now submit an OTR to provide treatment beyond the twelfth session.

f. *Time and session planning:* People in group psychotherapy need to have a commitment to the sessions. However, over the span of six weeks it is possible (even likely) that a person may miss a session. When you request additional sessions, the managed care company often simply counts the number of weeks (assuming once-a-week meetings).

Therefore, request more time than is needed for sessions. If the sessions were to begin the first week in February and last for six weeks until March 15th, ask them to extend the dates until the end of March. You will still only be approved for six sessions but this will save you from having to resubmit paperwork asking for a time extension should the person miss a session during the authorization time.

Once you have the information, see if you can accommodate the demands for paperwork and the financial remuneration. If the answer is yes, proceed with the application. Some companies have asked for application fees of $100.00. In such a case, you want to confer with your colleagues who already have worked with the company. Sometimes these requests are made by start-up companies that are not going to be around long enough for you to reap the rewards of such an investment.

Contact your insurance company directly about providing materials to the managed care company. Problems often arise when you try to serve as a middle person between the information the managed care company needs and the insurance company. You will most likely need to authorize your insurance company to send information to the various managed care companies.

Before you send your application, *photocopy every page of the document you are sending.* Send your application "Return Receipt Requested." A number of providers have complained that after completing an exhaustive application, the managed care companies have misplaced it. Validating it being delivered and having a complete copy of the application are two good ways to protect yourself.

Chapter 2

BASIC ACTION METHODS

The major contribution action methods bring to the interactive group therapy process is consciousness. Elevating participation in the group to include sensory modalities other than just verbalization allows participants to be more present, more aware, and as a consequence more conscious.

Consciousness is no small matter. It enhances our interactions by making them intentional. When action is added to the group process, it dissolves passivity. Acting on thoughts and feelings gives greater visibility to our inner world and greater energy to our words. Action also helps clarify our thoughts and feelings. When we act, we see our intentions more clearly than when we only use words or only reflect on our thoughts and feelings. This clarity comes as a result of internal and external feedback. This clarity then can be used to adjust our way of being.

Energy follows action. Adding action to your repertoire of clinical skills can be a natural step. Our need to talk, interact, and simply be with each other is part of our development as a species. Group psychotherapy is the most viable method for initiating, improving, and evaluating connections. Adding action techniques is a dramatic way to alter the process of a group. It focuses the consciousness of the members on their interactions, which in turn channels and enhances the energy within the group.

Perhaps one of the most common errors group facilitators make when they first begin using action methods is to have a group member engage in an encounter or rehearsal at the onset of the action. While it is certainly appropriate to use role-playing to rehearse a new behavior or to act out an encounter, it usually is not the best place to start. Doing so can result in distancing the member from the group (if he or she is not ready for such an event) or alienating members of the group who cannot relate to the encounter. Additionally, the member may be able to change his or her behavior in the group but, if not adequately supported, may be unable to carry over the newly learned behaviors into the outside environment. The solution to this dilemma may come from using the action method as a means of support. Creating an atmosphere of support is one of the most important contributions the facilitator can make to the group. If you are going to make an error, it is best to make it on the side of having too much support rather than too little. Trust and safety are the cornerstones of every group. When used at the right time, action methods can help create this ambiance for the group.

This chapter introduces, and invites you to experiment with, the most basic action techniques: the double, the empty chair, the use of an auxiliary, and role reversal. The greater portion of this chapter will be devoted to the double. It is the cornerstone of all the action methods and is perhaps the most valuable technique you will learn from this book.

THE DOUBLE

Jacob Moreno's contributions to the field of group psychotherapy are enormous (Moreno, 1946, 1947, 1951, 1956, 1978; Moreno & Moreno, 1959). He is credited with developing group psychotherapy as a treatment modality as well as having coined the phrase itself. Because of his invention of psychodrama and its many techniques, and his prolific contributions to the psychotherapy literature, Moreno has been hailed as the "psychiatrist of the century." However, of all his accomplishments, the creation of the *double* technique is perhaps his most valuable. If you adopt only one technique from this book, let it be the double. It is elegant in its simplicity and yet profoundly enlightening, moving, and helpful when done properly. The double has three purposes: (a) providing emotional support, (b) giving emotional expression, and (c) reorganizing perceptions.

You can do a great deal with the double. The technique is used when one person has presented a problem that is significant enough for exploration within the group. This person becomes the *protagonist*. The many parameters that determine the selection of the protagonist have been discussed elsewhere (Blatner, 1996; Tomasulo, 1992) and will be discussed again in Chapter 5. In most cases the protagonist presents a situation that reflects a deficiency or an interpersonal or intrapsychic conflict. This deficiency or conflict then becomes the central issue of the drama.

One or more other group members then are chosen as the double to speak out the feelings or experiences of the protagonist. The person playing the double mimics the protagonist in a way that gives clues to the protagonist's internal state. This exercise develops an *isomorphic* condition for the protagonist, which allows emotional expression, emotional support, and the reorganizing of perceptions to emerge. If the double can create an atmosphere in which the protagonist feels supported and understood, the opportunity for change is greatly enhanced.

The facilitator asks the double how he or she thinks the protagonist feels. The double speaks in the first person in order to reflect the protagonist's feeling state. The facilitator may have to cue the double to say "I feel ... " and then ask the double how he or she thinks the protagonist feels. In the beginning the facilitator may have to do this several times. The facilitator also may have to demonstrate how doubling is done. However, once doubling becomes part of the regular routine of the group, members will easily and spontaneously offer "I" statements.

The following vignette illustrates how to use a protagonist and a double within a session.

Case of Bernard and Martin. Bernard says, "I got a call from my brother and he was drunk again." As this issue is in keeping with the needs of the group, Bernard is invited to be the protagonist. He selects someone from the group he thinks might grasp how he felt. He chooses Martin, who then tries to identify Bernard's feelings. He might say, "I am very angry and sad when my brother calls me and is drunk" or "I am scared because my brother usually gets violent when he is drunk and I start worrying about what he might do" or "My whole family is so screwed up I wish they would just leave me alone."

Choosing the Double

The double can be chosen in one of several ways: (a) the facilitator can choose the double, (b) the protagonist can choose the double from the group, (c) a group member can volunteer, (d) the facilitator can do the doubling, or (e) the protagonist can double himself or herself. The double should be a person who understands the protagonist's thoughts and feelings. As stated above, the group facilitator can select a member of the group to double the feeling of the protagonist or a member in the group may volunteer to be the double; however, the most reliable conditions occur when the protagonist is allowed to select his or her own double. The protagonist will know best who to pick because of the *tele* (the natural connections between people) or the *transference* between the protagonist and the chosen double. (See Chapter 5.)

Doubles may be single, in pairs (to allow for contrast, amplification, or restatement) or in multiples (to help the protagonist experience acceptance or universality with fellow members).

Position of the Double

Typically, the double is positioned behind the protagonist and slightly to one side. The protagonist can be sitting or standing, and the double can assume the same physical stance as the protagonist. Assuming the same physical stance as the protagonist allows the double to "warm-up" to the internal state of the protagonist. Or, the protagonist can be seated and the double can stand behind his or her chair. The position behind the protagonist is symbolic of the supportive position of the parents. Our parents are the first people to think for us. We become who we are largely because of their influence. The position behind the protagonist is nonconfrontational and supportive.

The only *contraindication* for the position behind the protagonist is when it increases anxiety, as it usually does with people who are paranoid. In this case, the double may stand at the protagonist's side.

After the protagonist has presented his issue, he can move his chair into the middle of the group, or he can remain in his chair as part of the circle.

Multiple Doubles

A double, as said before, may be single, a pair, or multiple. A *multiple double* is used when it is necessary to create significant support for the protagonist. When several people come into the double role, the protagonist feels understood by the group in a direct way. Using a multiple double format activates *therapeutic factors* relevant to *acceptance, cohesion,* and *universality* within the group.

The protagonist presents his or her story and then asks who, in the group, understands how he or she feels. As members volunteer, the facilitator invites them to stand behind the protagonist and say the feelings they believe the protagonist would have in the situation described. It is important to check with the protagonist to make sure that what is being said "fits" with the protagonist's internal experience. If not, there may need to be a correction (see the section below on correcting the double). Once this is accomplished, the next group member is invited up, followed by the next, and so on.

In the earlier example, if Bernard had not chosen Martin as his double, and it was not immediately clear who the best double would be, then I would invite several people from the group to come stand behind him and say what they think he feels. Besides the range of statements offered earlier, other possibilities might emerge from the other doubles:

> "All I can think about when he calls is how I used to be when I got drunk."

> "I just want to hang up on him, but I don't. I feel so codependent."

> "I want to drink after he calls."

> "I wonder where the hell is the rest of my family? Why am I always the one he calls?"

> "He is such an idiot. I don't want anything to do with him."

Each of these statements may be a portion of what the protagonist is feeling. Some may be more accurate than others—and some may be wrong. In any case, there is now a significant array of feelings to be explored. The protagonist can select from those doubles the one (or two) to further his or her understanding in the situation. Once the double(s) have been chosen, they continue with the line of thinking they have just brought up. In this way, the depth of the support can be more readily experienced by the protagonist.

Paired Doubles

When doubles verbalize internal conflict, the protagonist experiences his or her struggle being understood by his or her peers. If the double is played by a pair (a *paired double*), you should have one person stand behind the protagonist to the left and one to the right. A group member can play one half of the pair, and the facilitator the other half, or two group members can play the double pair.

A pair can effectively reflect conflict situations and those wrought with ambivalence. To continue our previous example using a paired double:

> One of the pair says to Bernard, "My brother always bothers me. He is always calling me when he is drunk." The other adds, "I like it when my brother calls me when he is drunk. It makes me feel I am better off than him." One says, "I am angry that my brother called me." The other says, "I'm angry, but I am also afraid that my brother is going to hurt someone, maybe even me." Thus, two strong emotions, anger *and* fear, are expressed.

Reflecting the internal struggle back to the protagonist helps him become aware of the true nature of his feelings. If the conflict portrayed does not reflect the internal conflict, it can be corrected.

The Protagonist as His or Her Own Double

Playing one's own double offers the protagonist clarification, awareness, and acknowledgment. It also provides a model for others in the group when they double for the protagonist. When the protagonist acts as her own double, she reverses roles with the space behind her chair. In the role of her own double, the protagonist makes statements about her feelings, which the facilitator then asks her to amplify, restate, or alter in some way to enhance the clarity of the feeling. The protagonist can play his or her own double as a way of showing the group how he or she feels. If Bernard had raised the issue about his brother calling with little or no description of his feelings (e.g., "My brother called me drunk again last night"), I would first have had him play his own double. This would not have precluded other forms of doubling. After the protagonist has acted as his or her own double, it could be followed by a single, paired, or multiple double.

Correcting the Double

A double can be corrected in two primary ways. The double can adjust previously made statements once he or she realizes that they do not match the internal state of the protagonist, or the protagonist can reverse roles with the double to clarify the statements. When a double says something to the protagonist, the facilitator must check it out by saying something to the protagonist such as, "Does that sound right to you?" If the double has made an error, he or she can try to correct it with another statement.

In our case example, if Martin, as the double, said, "I am totally enraged by my brother calling me when he is drunk. He's got no respect for my privacy!" I would ask Bernard, "Is that how you feel?" If he agreed, we would move on. If not, and if Martin had no modification, I would ask Bernard to reverse roles with Martin and correct the statement. This *role reversal* would serve as a *role prescription* for Martin. They would then reverse roles back to their original positions, and Martin would repeat what Bernard had said. This ensures that the feelings are on target, as the protagonist himself identified them during the role reversal. In this way, the protagonist teaches others in the group what he or she is feeling, and the doubles are able to more accurately indicate feelings for the protagonist. Sometimes it is necessary to repeat the role reversal. It is important to remember that the people who are playing the double use *projection* to try to place themselves in the role. In doing this they, of course, run the risk of misunderstanding the protagonist's feelings. Correction through role reversal enables them to identify more accurately with the protagonist's feelings.

Practicing the Double

Practicing the role of the double can be a useful group exercise. Here are some guidelines:

1. Pair off with a person in the group you feel is mutually willing to work with you.

2. Choose who will go first as the protagonist and who will be the double.

3. As protagonist, think of a "peak experience" in your life, a time when you felt exceptionally good. Assume a body

posture or produce a physical action that conveys your joy and sense of well being. When you are ready, explain the situation and your reactions.

4. As the double, stand behind the protagonist and adopt the same body posture and movements. Try to draw on your own emotional experiences and imagine feeling how the protagonist feels.

5. Put words to your doubling. Use the first person, as if you were having the experience yourself (e.g., "I am feeling so good about what I have done. I've never quite felt like this. This is terrific!").

6. Check with the protagonist and adjust what you are saying to match what the protagonist says. For example, you as the double say, "This was the most profound experience of my life." The protagonist does not agree and says, "It was super—but not the most profound experience I have ever had." You then adjust your feedback to reflect this softening of intensity. Continue this process until the protagonist indicates that you have accurately matched the feeling.

7. Reverse roles and follow steps 3 through 6.

8. Once you have each practiced both roles, begin the exercise again, only this time, use a negative feeling or experience. Repeat steps 3 through 7.

9. After completing both positive and negative exercises, discuss what it felt like to play both roles. Identify the difficulties and the surprises you encountered. Note in particular what you liked about the exercise.

This practice experience can be done with just two participants and an observer or in the context of a whole group. If done in a group setting, the exercise should end when the entire group discussing the experience.

THE EMPTY CHAIR

The *empty chair*, a vacant chair is used to symbolize another person or role. This extraordinary technique is both simple and profound. It is one of the easiest and most dramatic methods to use. It is deceptively simple. A group member who has described a conflict or problem with a person in his or her life is asked to imagine that person in an empty chair. The member then is asked to tell that person how he or she feels by speaking to the chair. The protagonist can have a conversation with those who are unavailable to him or her. The deceased, God, spirit guides, unborn children, famous role models, future lovers, and many others can be imagined sitting in the empty chair. When encountering any of these projections, protagonists come to awareness, offer insights, and reveal character features that previously had gone unnoticed.

The empty chair can be used to deal with the following three conditions:

Interpersonal Conflict (External Conflicts),

Intrapsychic Conflict and an Observing Ego (Internal Conflicts), and

Past, Present, and Future Issues (Time Sensitive Factors).

The empty chair technique offers a glimpse of the projection of the protagonist. The individual with an interpersonal conflict projects his or her perception of the individual with whom he or she is in conflict into the empty chair. The value of this technique lies in the undiluted projection of feelings. How the protagonist has sized up the person in the interpersonal external conflict becomes apparent.

Setting the Scene

Setting the scene with an empty chair reveals the emotional ambiance. Asking "What chair would your mother sit in?" causes the protagonist to make decisions about his or her mother's personality that can paint a psychological portrait for the group. "She would sit in that chair. The only one that is different in the room. She liked drawing attention to herself. She would choose that chair because she would feel that it would make her stand out." Or, "She would pick the chair closest to the door. That way she could leave any time she wanted. She wouldn't have to be part of the group. She could excuse herself and slip out without having to make conversation." Choosing the chair begins the process of creating the role. Another question is, "How far away from you is she in the conversation?" This is a question about psychological distancing.

Role Reversal and the Empty Chair

The *gestalt* version of the empty chair technique, developed by Moreno, is a one-sided event that is not so much an *encounter* as an opportunity for *catharsis*. The protagonist simply expresses his or her feelings. This has obvious value but does not use the full therapeutic potential of the process. The encounter is more complete and the conflict is understood in a vastly different way when a role reversal with the empty chair is attempted. In this case, after expressing his or her feelings to the empty chair, the protagonist sits in the chair and speaks out the feelings of the person with whom he or she is in conflict. This enables the protagonist to gain insight into the other person's feelings and point of view.

Role reversal is an essential part of the empty chair technique for the following reasons.

First, having the protagonist sit in the empty chair and speak the feelings of the other changes his or her perceptual view of the situation. It helps the protagonist develop an empathic awareness of the other's role. The group also will understand at a concrete level what the protagonist is dealing with. As a result, they will be able to better appreciate and perhaps to relate to the protagonist's struggle. Often, people in the group will connect with something from the other person's reaction as enacted by the protagonist. This deepens the possibility that members will be drawn into the role-play. The encounter is more complete because both people in the conflict are represented.

Second, beyond the emotional empathy that can happen during role reversal, being in the role of the other actually helps with the need to separate self from other. When playing the role of the other person in the empty chair, protagonists realize that the person they are playing is *not* them. While this may seem obvious, it is nonetheless significant. The event of being the other allows a greater degree of separateness to evolve.

Third, reversing roles with the empty chair increases an alternative awareness of the situation. To carry on a conversation in your head between yourself and another is nowhere near as powerful as acting it out with an empty chair. You become liberated from the confines of the intellectual and rational features of your cognitive functioning. A more emotionally intuitive aspect of yourself is engaged in the act of actually becoming, not merely imagining, the other. Protagonists are usually astounded to hear themselves speak in the other role.

Case of Neal. Neal had had a string of relationships with women that started out with a high degree of intensity and hope, but soon deteriorated into extremely destructive antagonism. He was aware of the pattern that plagued him but was not able to change it in a meaningful way. Although fully aware of the pattern, he would act out the destructive features of the relationship. While it takes two to tango, and the problems his partners brought to the relationships were certainly important, Neal was the person in therapy and the one choosing these women. It was his self-defeating pattern that we could investigate. In an empty chair exercise, Neal sat across from his latest antagonistic partner. He said how he felt, expressed his anger, yelled, blamed, criticized, and in short, vented his feelings.

If we had left the use of the empty chair there, it would have had some benefit. A catharsis can drain out excess emotions and allow a different way of thinking about the situation to emerge. Or, at the least, the tension the protagonist is experiencing is released in a manner that reduces stress and anxiety.

However, Neal was asked to play his partner. He was incredulous. "What, are you kidding? You want me to play her? No way. All she is going to do is pick on me. I don't want to do that." Neal started laughing as he said these words. "I guess I have some strong feelings about this." He laughed again and went over into the other seat.

"I don't know what you want." This was the first thing Neal said in the role reversal being his girlfriend. He stayed in her role and continued, "You always give me double messages. I never know when you are happy, or when you are going to get angry. You make me so nervous because all I want to do is please you. But then you give me a double message. You tell me on Monday that we're going out on Saturday night. I don't hear from you the rest of the week because you are too busy. Then Saturday comes and (now Neal is yelling) I STILL DON'T HEAR FROM YOU. I CALL AND LEAVE A MESSAGE ON YOUR MACHINE AND YOU DON'T RETURN MY CALL UNTIL FIVE MINUTES TO TEN SATURDAY NIGHT. I tell you that I am ready for bed and in my pajamas, and you throw a shit fit because you say you told me we were going out. You keep testing me, Neal, and I keep trying to pass the test, but you are determined to make me fail. I can't win. I can't get it right with you. Why should I try? Why should I try?"

When Neal got back into his own chair, he was stunned. He was speechless. Neal learned for the first time that he was at the root of the problem. His treatment of her, from her perspective, was nothing short of abusive. He never had understood his behavior in this way before. This was a turning point for Neal, and he now was able to use his awareness to bring about positive changes in his behavior.

Case of Karen. Karen was severely sexually abused by her father. After a sufficient time in the group, when she was able to trust me and the other members, she allowed herself to play the role of her father. She had resisted playing this role for a long time because she thought it was "too disgusting" and "too horrible" to do. Finally, one evening she allowed herself to play the role of her father. He was truly evil in her role-play: seductive, lewd, and narcissistic. "He" revealed his character and his own pathology to the group.

When Karen returned to her seat, she was empowered by the realization that her father was truly abusive and that she was not responsible for what had happened. Additionally, she realized that she had free will as to how she could respond to the memories of her father. In technical terms, she was aware that the introject of her father did not have to become her vision of herself. She had been mortally afraid she would become like her father because he was the sole influence in her childhood life. During her role-play of him, she became aware that she was separate from him and that she was the one who could determine how she wanted to be. This was a startling and powerful shift for Karen. She knew it intellectually, but *feeling* it in the drama made a big difference in her understanding of herself. She was able to complete the empty chair exercise back in her own role and chair feeling more empowered and decidedly more assertive.

Practicing the Empty Chair and Role Reversal

This exercise is designed to help you understand the mechanics of using the empty chair. It is not intended for deep psychological evaluation. It can be done alone or in a group.

1. Choose a person from history, mythology, your past or future, religion, or fantasy that you would like to ask a question. For the purpose of the exercise, choose a per-

son or entity and a question that are not too disturbing or negative.

2. Place an empty chair in front of you as far away or as close as you want this person or entity to be.

3. Stand or sit in a place that represents the right emotional distance for you and ask your question.

4. Once the question has been asked, reverse roles and sit in the empty chair and answer.

5. Continue this dialogue until you feel you can safely end the conversation.

6. Take a moment to reflect on what was gathered from this experience. If you are alone you may want to write your reactions in your journal. If you are working as part of a group exercise, discuss your individual reactions collectively.

AN AUXILIARY

The use of an *auxiliary* combines elements of the double, the empty chair, and role reversal. In this technique, the protagonist chooses an auxiliary rather than an empty chair, and then reverses roles with the auxiliary. The auxiliary, like the double, is chosen on the basis of transference or tele. This means that the person being chosen for the auxiliary role identified by the protagonist brings some dynamic presence to the encounter. This is the major difference between the use of an auxiliary and the use of an empty chair. The empty chair is employed when you want to minimize the protagonist's reactions to a stimulus (an auxiliary). It gives the protagonist a greater amount of control and is generally thought to be less threatening than using an auxiliary. The use of an auxiliary on the other hand amplifies the encounter and creates a more interactional dynamic. This is due to the fact that the protagonist has to contend with another human being (the auxiliary), who naturally will activate his or her own defenses and reactions.

CONDITIONS FOR USING THE METHODS

Our discussion so far has focused on using action methods to deal with issues relating to interpersonal conflict (or, external conflicts). These techniques are also effective with intrapsychic conflict (or, internal conflicts), and past, present, and future issues (or, time-sensitive factors).

Intrapsychic Conflict (Internal Conflict)

Intrapsychic conflict represents a division within the self. This division of thought can lead to indecision, anxiety, and even depression. To role-play this condition, the protagonist begins by arranging two chairs in a way that symbolizes the conflict. They may be opposite one another, they may be perpendicular to one another, they may be as far apart in the room as is physically possible. This symbolic arrangement sets the tone for the intrapsychic encounter. The protagonist begins in one chair speaking from the one side of the intrapsychic conflict. Once this has been accomplished, the protagonist reverses roles and sits in the chair representing the other point of view. In this way the internal dialogue is externalized. In doing so, the drama takes on the property of something that can change, that can be modified.

At this point you may wish to introduce auxiliaries to enhance the role-play. This can be done in several different ways. The following are some possibilities:

1. Have the protagonist (or you as facilitator) choose an auxiliary (or have one volunteer) to play one side of the internal conflict. This gives the protagonist the opportunity to cope with this position in an overt way that often leads to new insights.

2. Have the protagonist (or you as facilitator) choose one auxiliary (or have one volunteer) to play *both* sides of the conflict. In this way the protagonist gets to witness *one* person struggle with both sides of the encounter from an observer's point of view. This observation often provides

a fresh perspective on the internal struggle for the protagonist and may help develop the protagonist's *observing ego*.

3. Have the protagonist (or you as facilitator) choose two auxiliaries (or have two volunteer) to play each side of the conflict. This is a very powerful way for the protagonist to observe the internal struggle. The protagonist then can experiment with changing the way these two voices relate to one another. The protagonist can script for the two auxiliaries a new dialogue between each other and then can witness the efficacy of the new approach. This becomes a helpful tool for the protagonist to change his or her way of dealing with the conflict.

4. Have the protagonist begin by stating one position in one chair. Then invite other members of the group to double for that position. This use of a multiple double allows each position to be fully explored in terms of supportive elements, ulterior motives, and unspoken features that may not have been elaborated on by the protagonist. The protagonist then would take the conflicting role in the other chair, followed again with multiple doubling. In doing this, the balance between these perspectives may shift, giving the protagonist a greater awareness of each perspective.

5. As the facilitator, you may provide a modified version of the above by doubling for both perspectives, playing an auxiliary, or perhaps even playing both auxiliaries. While this approach is viable, it offers the least amount of interaction between members of the group and as such should be considered a less desirable alternative.

Past, Present, and Future Issues (Time-Sensitive Factors)

Often group members struggle with dilemmas that are encased in specific time periods. They may feel trapped by the past, anxious about the future, or stuck in the present. In these instances, the empty chair technique used in a time-related enactment will be helpful.

To begin, the protagonist sets an empty chair somewhere in the room where he or she feels he or she is at the present time. Next, the protagonist places chairs where his or her past and future selves are in relationship to the present. Again, the protagonist can use the empty chairs to act out each of the roles.

Another alternative is to use auxiliaries who learn how to play the roles from the protagonist. In this case, the protagonist reverses roles with the empty chair and gives a sample, a *role prescription* if you will, to the auxiliary who is to play the role in question. In this way you have the best of both worlds. You have the protagonist reverse roles with the empty chair, followed by the empty chair being replaced by an auxiliary. This is a very powerful way for protagonists to view their current status. For example, a protagonist might choose to put the "past" chair very close behind while having the "future" relatively far away from the "present" chair. Then the role of the "past" can be used to provide a script of what that role represents. This role prescription would then allow another member of the group (now called an auxiliary) to take on the "past" role in that chair, while the protagonist returns to the "present" chair. In this fashion, the setting has been set for the protagonist to have a dialogue with the auxiliary in the "past" chair. During this dialogue, it would be important to have the protagonist reverse roles with the auxiliary when significant questions are being asked. This allows the protagonist to encounter his or herself in a dialogue with the past.

Chapter 3

THERAPEUTIC FACTORS

Therapeutic factors are the components of therapy that are beneficial to the patients or clients. In group therapy, they emerge during the group process and are the result of actions by the group facilitator, the members, and the group as a whole. Irving Yalom (1975) listed 11 of these factors. Students of his have added a few of their own.

This chapter describes 14 therapeutic factors that cover a wide range of interactive behaviors and conditions. These factors are:

1. Acceptance/cohesion
2. Universality
3. Altruism
4. Installation of hope
5. Guidance
6. Catharsis
7. Modeling
8. Self-understanding

9. Interpersonal action

10. Self-disclosure

11. Corrective recapitulation of the primary family

12. Existential factors

13. Imparting of information (education)

14. Social skills development

Generally speaking, the more these factors are present in a group, the more therapeutic the group is. The facilitator has the job of activating these factors. Of all the therapeutic duties the facilitator must perform, ensuring the emergence of therapeutic factors is the most important.

A facilitator creates these factors in many different ways. In some instances, a simple acknowledgment that a factor (like altruism) has occurred is sufficient. Other times, the facilitator must be more direct and concretely help members label what they have learned (like self-understanding). In still other instances, the facilitator may need to play a very direct, supportive role in bringing about a therapeutic factor (like catharsis).

ACCEPTANCE/COHESION

Members feel a sense of belonging and being valued by each other. This sense of being connected is fostered by positive interactions. Trusting others and being safe are usually central to feeling accepted. However, a sense of cohesion sometimes can follow from a negative encounter.

Case of Joan and Helena. These group members were antagonistic toward one another. Their opposition was regular and, at times, intense. The group had difficulty dealing with their direct verbal aggression toward each other and their encounters required a significant degree of facilitation. Through the use of action methods (the double, the auxiliary, and role reversal), both

Joan and Helen were able to recognize their transferential relationship with one another. Over time they were finally able to acknowledge the core reason for their disharmony. Each reflected the despised self of the other. In finally acknowledging this, they were able to see their reactions as projections that needed to be assimilated and understood. The group followed this process, and it set the stage for others to work through their issues in encountering the despised self through transferences with others.

In this case, the acceptance and cohesion factor was activated by strong negative encounters that ultimately were resolved in the group. The working through process allowed group members to share an experience that enhanced their development.

Joan and Helen were able to experience their conflict with one another in the group environment because it was safe. Each felt accepted by the group and, as a result, they were able not only to express their negative feelings for one another but also to assimilate the origin of their projections. The group was able to witness their encounter and see that differences can have an insightful, positive outcome. This adds to the cohesion of the group and fosters future work between individuals. Members are left feeling that they are accepted by others in the group, and that the membership in the group provides a safe vehicle for personal work to be done.

UNIVERSALITY

The common acknowledgment of a shared experience by group members is referred to as universality.

Universality occurs when members of the group have experienced a similar phenomenon or when a feeling is universally understood. In a women's group one member discussed the dehumanizing and painful experience of having a mammography. Her feelings were echoed by others in the group. It is not uncommon that one therapeutic factor gives way to another. In this case, the universality of the group ushered in the feeling of acceptance by the member relating her story.

> **Case of Ellen.** In a specialized group for people with mild and moderate mental retardation, Ellen spoke of the humiliation of being called "retarded" by children waiting for the school bus. The moment Ellen mentioned this, she began to cry. The other members began to shake their heads and immediately offered her their stories of similar experiences. The support and understanding she felt during this exchange of information was possible only from people who had had the same experience. Without this experience, others could sympathize. But those in the group knew what Ellen was saying in a different way.

ALTRUISM

Members spontaneously help others in the group. This helping is usually unsolicited and is the result of a spontaneous, unselfish desire to be of assistance. Helping others without the need to have that help reciprocated is the cornerstone of altruism. What makes altruism a particularly powerful therapeutic factor is that one act of altruism by one person inspires others' altruistic acts.

Altruism is perhaps the most easily recognizable factor and the simplest for a facilitator to acknowledge. Passing tissues to a member who is crying or bringing in a self-help book for another member going through a similar situation are common examples.

> **Case of Enrico.** Enrico was in an anger management group for men and women. The trigger for Enrico was strong emotions. If he saw his girlfriend cry it would activate him and he would have an outburst. Over time he had become more aware of the physiological arousal

that accompanied his anger and was gaining greater control over his reactions. In one session, he sat next to a woman who related a situation in her life that made her cry. As she was crying Enrico was noticeably upset and uncomfortable. As the crying continued Enrico excused himself from the room and returned with a box of tissues. This spontaneous act of altruism was instantly noticed by others in the group as a hallmark of his emotional development. Again, the emergence of this therapeutic factor gave way to another one: instillation of hope.

INSTALLATION OF HOPE

Over time, positive changes will occur in people's lives as a result of having worked through an issue in the group. Additionally, they will have had the opportunity to report on positive events in their life or situations with which they have learned to cope. Witnessing this growth, other members in the group gain a sense of hope regarding their own condition. Rarely would everyone in a group be at a low point in their coping skills. The variety of members' abilities allows for some degree of optimism and hope to be circulating within most groups.

The same women's group mentioned in the example for universality eventually had a member who was struggling with a recent diagnosis of breast cancer. The women in the group who had had similar diagnoses and treatment shared their experiences. Members discussed and evaluated local resources and engaged in a rich discussion of treatment options, which gave the individual significant hope in coping with her condition.

GUIDANCE

Members receiving guidance from members is sometimes helpful but difficult to facilitate adequately. In most groups, direct advice is not tolerated or useful. In the large majority of instances, advice-giving is not helpful and is often infuriating to the person receiving the advice. The more effective type of guidance a person can get is from other people sharing their experience.

Case of Barbara. A divorced woman, Barbara, who was having some difficulty with her ex-husband, was given some specific information about what to do and how to deal with the situation by Diane. The advice was particular to the situation, and Diane was empathic in her delivery of the information. This advice, although good, was not being accepted by Barbara. The facilitator made this type of advice more palatable by asking Diane how she knew this. "How is it that you know exactly what to do?" Diane revealed her own story. This information now became a sharing. Diane gave Barbara advice *based on her experience*.

Advice filtered through the experience of the advice giver is much less confrontive. The person receiving the information can accept or reject the sharing as he or she feels relevant. Thus, the person receiving the information can filter it based on personal experience. Simultaneously, the advice giver can offer information without having the burden of trying to make it fit the other person's view.

CATHARSIS

The purging of emotions has been a central feature in the therapeutic factors offered by psychotherapy since its inception. Individual or group catharsis may occur. Purging can be positively or negatively charged. Many theories exist as to what allows a catharsis to occur but will not be discussed here. I will note, however, that the benefit of this therapeutic factor is not limited to the person having the catharsis. Witnessing it can mediate a positive change in other members' personal growth.

Case of Maureen. Maureen had significant issues with her alcoholic father. Talking to her father in a role-play about her disappointments, she became quite agitated and angry. After reversing roles and speaking from her father's part, she came back into her role and began to cry. The role reversal had made her aware of her father's inability to understand her needs. Her anger was replaced by a profound sense of grief at the loss of the illusion that her father would be able to respond to her adequately. Her weeping had the power of authenticity and relevance to other members. What followed was a deep sharing by other members of their coming to grips with the inadequacy of being understood by significant others in their own lives. Many members also were able to share how they had coped with similar realizations.

MODELING

Other than our own efforts, nothing has more impact on us than watching others struggle with pertinent issues in their lives. When group members witness others develop (either through watching a role-play or by listening to them relate an experience), they learn from these observations through a form of identification. The use of modeling through role-playing is particularly good in enhancing vicarious learning.

Case of Artie. When Artie watched Sam enact a drama with his ex-wife, he saw how Sam was drawn into a conflict, then "baited" into acting out. During the drama a member of the group doubled for Sam's wife and said, "I chose you because I needed someone to act out my anger for me. I can't do it, and if I can get you to go off, you can be angry enough for both of us." Artie saw this for the first time as a representation of his own marriage. Through Sam's model, Artie gained insight into his own relationship.

SELF-UNDERSTANDING

Members learn something important about themselves through feedback from others in the group. On occasion, the feedback may be confrontational yet constructive. Even when feedback is uncomfortable, it may be accepted in the interest of gaining some insight about one's self.

Case of Artie. To follow up from the example of Sam and Artie, Artie began to understand the mechanics of how he would take on his wife's anger and display it. This insight led to feedback from members in the group, who saw Artie as a sponge for other people's anger. Members gave him specific feedback of times in the group when he had taken on the outrage he felt another member should be feeling. Often this was followed by Artie getting angry "for" the other person. This type of self-understanding was very helpful for Artie. Perhaps for the first time in his life he became more fully conscious of the dynamics that drove much of his anger.

INTERPERSONAL ACTION

Learning takes place as a by-product of trying to adapt to and relate constructively to the group. The group format offers a structure within which the group norms are set and members can learn through interaction how best to accommodate to the norms.

Case of Jake. Jake had been in a group for several months when he got his first taste of interpersonal learning. He was always ready with a kind word or a simple, canned explanation ("Everything happens for a reason," "Let go and let God," "Thanks for sharing"). Group members eventually confronted Jake, telling him that, rather than supportive and helpful, they found his involvement inauthentic, insincere, and an indication of his shallowness. Initially, Jake was offended, defending his statements as attempts to be involved and helpful. The group members who confronted him pointed out that his statements kept him from sharing about his own life rather than involving him. They kept him from self-disclosure and from relating at a deeper level with the group.

Jake was astonished by this feedback—but, at the same time, he was not unfamiliar with it. Over the years other people had repeatedly said similar things to him. Ultimately group members said they had come to discount what Jake said, seeing it as trivializing and insincere. They simply did not trust him because his responses were so shallow. This feedback provided Jake with interpersonal learning that allowed him to make changes in the way he interacted, self-disclosed, and related to members in the group. Eventually he was able to change his interactions with people both in and out of the group.

SELF-DISCLOSURE

Self-disclosure is the revealing of one's feelings, thoughts, and facts about oneself. Two types of self-disclosure can be observed in the group: horizontal and vertical. *Horizontal self-disclosure* refers to less emotionally charged interpersonal exchanges. *Vertical self-disclosure* refers to personal information of greater emotional depth. Vertical self-disclosure by one member can activate self-disclosure of others. However, too much self-disclosure too soon by a member may cause that member to feel vulnerable and other members in the group to feel inhibited.

Jake Revisited. Continuing from the previous example, over the next several meetings Jake began to shift from shallow interactions (horizontal self-disclosures) to more personally involved types of sharing. He began to talk about how he was never validated for his feelings in his family of origin. He had learned in his family that it was safer to say little or something innocuous than to risk sharing something of meaning. These expressions of sharing were well received by the group, who felt they came to know him better. By shifting from a "safe" horizontal form of self-disclosure to one with greater depth and meaning, Jake changed his pattern of interaction in the group.

CORRECTIVE RECAPITULATION
OF THE PRIMARY FAMILY

Corrective recapitulation of the primary family is a therapeutic factor that generally refers to the ability of a member to work through feelings established in the family of origin and come to a corrective understanding of those feelings within the group. It may be that the level of trust and safety within the group, which is different from members' families of origin, is what allows for therapeutic change to take place. People are able to act in the group differently from how they can act in their families. The developed sense of trust and safety allow each member to try new behaviors that will promote positive changes.

Perhaps there is no greater therapeutic factor than that of corrective recapitulation of the primary family. Over time, members are likely to unconsciously reenact their roles from their family of origin. The most fascinating aspect of this phenomenon is that the acting out happens for each member simultaneously. Each member is embroiled in reenacting his or her role while other members are seeing the group as their own family! This accounts for how one person's behavior in the group is subject to multiple interpretations and reactions from different members.

Case of Ralph. Ralph was reluctant to reveal to the group that he was gay. He thought members would reject him, ask him to leave the group, make fun of him, or even physically assault him. When Ralph did reveal that he was gay, the group accepted his disclosure without negative reaction and acknowledged his concerns and courage. Ralph was taken aback by this and began to discuss the reasons for his hesitation. Ultimately he told what had happened when he had told his family. His father had assaulted him and his mother told him to move out. His brother had ridiculed Ralph and also assaulted him. Remarkably, Ralph had not realized that his inhibition was directly, almost verbatim, tied to his family of origin. When he revealed to the group who he was, the group provided a corrective experience for him. He was able to act in the group in a way that was different and better than in his family.

EXISTENTIAL FACTORS

The common bonds of inevitable death, loneliness, and suffering are shared by group members.

When collectively experienced in a group, this factor allows people to realize ultimate universality and consequent bonding. Unfortunately, this therapeutic factor is used as an all-encompassing determinant by Yalom to describe the type of bonding that takes place from this realization. This is most likely due to Yalom's orientation as an existentialist. What is more common, but not officially noted as a therapeutic factor, is a nonreligiously officiated spirituality to which many members in groups relate.

Consider the largest form of group process in the world: 12-step groups. These groups operate worldwide, with millions of members organized under a spiritual yet nonreligious process. The bonding that helps make change possible is not simply the realization that, as finite human beings, we have certain common bonds; rather, it is the realization that spiritual development through interaction and community with others can restore one's mental health. A lack of spirituality as a therapeutic factor may reflect the more traditional separation between science and religion. However, I believe we will arrive at a more inclusive understanding of how people make a therapeutic shift once researchers and clinicians add spirituality to their list of therapeutic factors found in groups.

> **Case of Charlie.** Charlie had been a group member for three years when he died unexpectedly. Members of the group were stunned by his death and began to discuss the uncertainties of life, the inescapability of death, and the need to "seize the day." Following this, group members made note of how important the group was in their lives and how each of them had been influenced by Charlie's participation.

IMPARTING OF INFORMATION
(EDUCATION)

The *imparting of information (education)* is the didactic element of group therapy. In groups dealing with specific topics—such as anger management, AIDS awareness, sex education, or advocacy—specific information on the topic may be introduced. The warm-up, enactment, and sharing then follow from this orientation.

At the first session of a group for people living with a someone who abuses drugs, the facilitator distributed a checklist of "codependent" behaviors. The list provided a definition and a detailed description of behaviors that "enabled" the substance abuser to maintain his or her level of addiction. These descriptions soon gave way to self-disclosures, which helped the members of the group become more cohesive. Again, we see how one therapeutic factor can bring about the emergence of other therapeutic factors.

SOCIAL SKILLS DEVELOPMENT

Social skills development refers to the immediate feedback available to group members through their social interactions in the group.

> **Case of Justin.** Justin frequently would yawn, fidget with his watch, tap his feet, and appear to drift off when others in the group talked. When confronted with his apparent lack of attention, Justin responded that he had been unaware he was disengaging from the group through his behavior. The facilitator encouraged Justin to find ways to relate to what was being said instead of simply being so self-absorbed. By working on his attention skills, Justin ultimately was able to experience interpersonal learning through feedback from other members of the group. He gained insight into his self-absorbtion and made changes in how he conducted himself both in and out of group.

PRACTICING RECOGNIZING
THERAPEUTIC FACTORS

1. Attend an open fellowship meeting of a 12-step group in your area. (Have a colleague join you, if possible, to help you process afterward what you witnessed.) Note the therapeutic factors that have emerged in the group. Following the group, identify the situation where you feel one of the therapeutic factors emerged and discuss this with your colleague. Respond to these questions:

   a. Would you have expected more of these factors to have emerged than you witnessed? Why or why not?

   b. Do you think there are more therapeutic factors present in a homogeneous group rather than a heterogeneous group?

   c. Are there ways to stimulate therapeutic factors if you are the facilitator of a group? What are some of your ideas?

   Stimulating the emergence of therapeutic factors should be an inherent goal for any facilitator. Therapeutic factors are features of a group that tend to evolve naturally when groups of people get together. As such, the collective, additive experience of these factors in an environment designed to enhance their presence and proliferation is the work of the facilitator.

   In general, action methods provide concrete vehicles for the activation and enhancement of therapeutic factors. In the previous chapter we talked about a multiple double. Consider how effective a multiple double can be in generating acceptance/cohesion, universality, installation of hope, or self-understanding. The action of having various members double for a protagonist provides a focus that will initiate or reinforce these factors.

  d. Do large groups encourage or inhibit the presence of therapeutic factors?

2. If you are part of a self study group, create a *fish bowl* where some of the members of the group take an active role in a group process while the remainder of the group observes and records therapeutic factors as they emerge. Follow this procedure for a period of one-half to one hour, then return to the full group and have the observers report their findings. Following this, members of the active group within the fish bowl discuss their experience. During this time, it is important to note interventions by the facilitator that have enhanced the emergence of therapeutic factors and those that may have inhibited them.

Chapter 4

ACTION METHODS IN USE: AN EXAMPLE

The following is a transcript from an actual group psychotherapy training session held for the purpose of training members in the use of psychodrama and sociodrama. The session took place on January 19, 1996. Certain phrases and identifying factors, as well as names, have been changed to preserve the identity of participants. Some editorial changes have been introduced to make the flow of the narrative easier to read. However, nothing substantive was altered. Each member of the group had the opportunity to review and approve of the transcript prior to publication. Analysis of the transcript as well as processing comments are introduced as Notes.

The seating arrangement for this session was as follows:

Don   Betsy

Catherine   Valerie

Melanie   Ted

Facilitator

65

The facilitator is a man, and the group begins with the facilitator asking about matters left over from the previous meeting held two weeks prior. The training group meets twice a month.

Facilitator: So, how about leftovers from last time?

Betsy: I haven't been the same since.

Facilitator: Ah, great!

Betsy: Not because of what happened here, but because of what Melanie said to me. She asked me about why I don't wear a wedding band. Well I don't even think about it. I mean, it's something I don't even give any thought to. And what has happened these past two weeks has been the rage and anger inside of me that has come up these past two weeks. It bothers me, and, well, I've had therapy and I thought to myself, "Gee, I addressed these issues." But I don't know, it just seemed to bring everything back up. It brought all that stuff back up, and I don't ... I just distance at home and I just want to be left alone. I can't seem to sort it all out. So that's what happened to me.

Facilitator: How did you move through that? How did you move through that experience?

Betsy: I haven't.

Facilitator: So you are still very much with it.

Betsy: Very angry. Because, there again, a lot of what happened had to do, there again, with his kids. I mean anything, anytime we have any problems, it has to do with his kids. And then, on top of that, he went there on Monday. And of course the holidays were crazy, and I never know what's going on. I don't know anything when it comes to that, where he's going. And I guess it brought up so much pain. There's so much pain around that period of time. It's just rage. Just a lot of rage inside of me. A horrible rage inside of me, and I've been with it. I don't know what to do. I don't know what to do. In fact I was half-tempted to call the person I was seeing [a therapist], and it's unusual because I usually do when I get stuck on something, but I haven't called her this time. I'm saying, "Well I've already dealt with these issues, or at least tried to deal with them, why is all this stuff coming up again?"

Facilitator: Yes, right.

Betsy: And that's what bothers me. Why is all this stuff coming up again?

Facilitator: How about others? Leftovers or new things?

Note: The facilitator in the beginning of the group is searching for themes and potential protagonists. Once a person has identified his or her issue or situation, the task is to gather input from others. This is the *warm-up* stage and is designed to help the members of the group get ready to interact with one another. The primary task of the facilitator is to create a safe and trusting atmosphere for the group to explore their issues. The work during this phase of the group is threefold:

1. *Invite* each participant to share what it is he or she may need to work on. This may come in the form of "leftovers" from the week before or new issues that may have come up in the interim. It includes interpersonal interactions that need to be dealt with between members in the group.

2. *Determine* whose issue or what theme would be most appropriate for the group to work on. If there is a universal theme, it may be appropriate to do a group exercise.

If one person's issues are able to attract the attention of the rest of the group, the facilitator may choose him or her as a protagonist. There are four ways to choose a protagonist:

a. the facilitator can choose a protagonist,

b. the group can choose a protagonist (through sociometry, see Chapter 5),

c. the protagonist can volunteer to work in the group, or

d. the protagonist can emerge from the work of another protagonist. This usually happens later in the group and is referred to as a "spin-off."

3. *Prevent* a protagonist from working in the group if there is not sufficient support for either the protagonist or the issue. To allow someone to work when there is insufficient support would be counterproductive.

Don: *(directed toward Betsy)* I don't know if it's a pertinent observation or not, but I just noticed to myself, coming into the room, that your face, to me, not knowing you very well and all, that you looked a lot different from last time. That you looked all shut down and suppressed last week. I don't doubt that this rage and whatever is still coming up, but your face now seems more peaceful and your eyes brighter, to me.

Melanie: I saw it, too.

Catherine: I saw it, too.

Facilitator: It looks like a lot of folks are nodding their heads about that. *(The people who were nodding their heads exaggerate their movements and everyone starts laughing.)*

Note: This is an example of *interpersonal learning*. Betsy is receiving feedback about how she is present in the group. The other members are telling her something she may not have been aware of.

Melanie:	It's funny, I have a good friend who is seeing a therapist, and she's dealing with issues, childhood issues, and she is going to write a letter to her dad, her dad's been dead a while, and I did all that. And she asked me if she could read my letter that I wrote to my father, and I found it yesterday, and I took it out and I read it to myself. And you're saying, and I kept asking, "How many times do we have to work through these issues?" But, you know, it just didn't touch me. Every other time I read it, I used to sit down and cry and just feel in here (*touches her heart*) the heartache from when I wrote it. And yesterday I just read it and I went "whew!" I can't believe I've been in such a good place, I'm almost afraid, I can't believe, it's too good. (*Everyone laughs.*)

Note: This is an illustration of *installation of hope*. As Melanie is talking, other members in the group are able to note that things can get better, and that Melanie is feeling the positive effects of the changes in her life.

Melanie:	It really is so wonderful. Every day is a gift. I am so grateful for everything, and I just can't believe that. I try to help a couple of other friends that I have who are having some problems: "Say it as many times as you need to. Deal with it as many times as you have to until ... " I guess with your description (*turns her attention toward the facilitator*) of the drop of water. I liked that.

Note: Melanie is referring to an analogy of the changes we experience in therapy as being like changing the color of water in a bucket by adding a new color drop by drop.

Facilitator: That the color of the water doesn't change with one or two drops. That it takes some time.

Melanie: Yeah. It just happens. I did Raki with a girlfriend of mine, and the energy between us was incredible. It has been just wonderful.

Don: You can see the transformation since last time.

Melanie: For both of us. *(to Betsy)* So keep doing it. And keep doing it, and keep doing it, and keep doing it.

Catherine: I have a request. I noticed, I got a flyer about the psychodrama conference in New York and I noticed you're [the facilitator] doing the *Course in Miracles* psychodrama, and I was wondering if sometime can we do one here?

Facilitator: Terrific.

Catherine: I'd like to do that here and see how you do that.

Facilitator: Sure. I'd like to see how I do it too. *(Everyone laughs.)*

Catherine: I don't know if I'll get to New York.

Facilitator: Sure. Actually it would be good, if it fits in with our schedule. I'll try to do it in February as a warm-up for the conference. That way, I've run it, I guess, half a dozen times, and I've modified it in different ways. I tried it one way, then cut and pasted, changed a few things. So it would be very helpful for me to bring it in. And we don't have to do the whole group on it. We can do it in the beginning of the group. Then you can see it, see how it works and what it evolves into. Yeah, I'll bring that in.

Melanie: I've also been thinking that I'd like to do a warm-up using the mandalas like the one we did in class.

Facilitator: Great.

Melanie: I don't know that I want to go on. Once everybody does their mandalas, I could just explain what it is and flip it back over to you [the facilitator]. *(Everyone laughs.)*

Facilitator: Wow.

Melanie: I've really been looking a lot at my artwork and thinking that it's been good for me.

Facilitator: Would you want to work in conjunction with somebody? You would do the warm-up and they would do the action?

Melanie: Sure, sure.

Facilitator: So you may want to think about when you might want to do that.

Melanie: Okay.

Facilitator: And who you might want to do that with, because I think that's a good way for us to work together.

Melanie: If somebody else is interested in artwork, interpreting artwork. Anybody.

Ted: Did you say mandala?

Melanie: Mandala. It's a circle. It's the Sanskrit word for circle.

Ted: I remember a book from so many years ago. I looked at it but I don't know anything about it.

Melanie: Jung has used the mandala.

Ted: I could bring it in.

Melanie: I'd like that.

Ted: I remember it as an interesting book. I like the pictures. I like the colors. I think I still have it.

Melanie: That would be great.

Don: I'd be interested.

Ted: I would like to bring it in because I really don't know anything about it, and I would like to learn more about it.

Melanie: Thanks.

Note: This is an example of spontaneous acts of *altruism.*

Facilitator: So, great, maybe we can pick a time and a date for that. So, you two might want to get together later on and discuss how you want to do the warm-up and then see how you want to structure the session.

Melanie: Okay.

Facilitator: That would be terrific.

Melanie: Okay.

Catherine: You know last week you *(talking to Betsy)* were talking about your daughter who has cancer, and I've had a tumor in my uterus for years now, and it's this big *(uses her hands to make a ball shape about the size of a grapefruit and starts laughing),* and I wonder why my stomach is sticking out now. But it's like this big and it's beginning to hurt a little bit now, so I thought I would go to the doctor. And I have avoided having it taken out because I don't have health insurance because if I had gotten any they wouldn't have paid for this because it's a preexisting condition. So I went to the doctor the other day. I had a flyer at home that I had saved for a couple of years and just kept it aside.

And most doctors said, "This thing is so huge that we are going to have to cut you open from side to side and remove this thing." And I'm like, that's six weeks recovery being out of my practice, and a week in the hospital with no hospitalization, so, uh, just let it go. But it bothered me. Ever since you talked about your daughter, this thing has been bothering me.

I took the flyer and I went to this doctor [mentions the doctor and facility in a nearby town]. And this doctor is one of 5% of doctors in this county that do laparoscopy, and he is going to take it out on the thirtieth.

He said, "I haven't had a challenge in my life for quite a while, so I guess this is my challenge." And I'm like, "Okay!" And I am so happy that there are doctors like that.

He said he will "operate at eight in the morning and, if you're okay, you can go home at eight at night." He did everything he could to keep the cost down. "You don't need this admission test, you don't need that one, you don't need that one." And he was really, really caring. It is such a miracle. So, hopefully I'll be here on the second, but if I'm not, don't do the *Course in Miracles*!

Facilitator: *(joking)* Don't do the *Course in Miracles*.

Catherine: Until I come! And for some reason I am not even that worried about it. It's such a miracle that I got the right doctor there, and he is such a caring doctor. I said, "What do you charge?" and he said, "I don't know." And I said, "You sound like me!" *(Everyone laughs.)*

So I'm happy about that and I'm not even nervous. And they'll take me to [a local, but less well known hospital] for follow-up care. I called my old doctor. He said, "There is no way anyone can take that out without cutting you open." And I said, "Yes there is!" And losing my uterus is such a central part of being a woman, but that doesn't really bother me. And my mom is back and she had another operation, but she is still in pain and is going to the doctor today to find out what's wrong with her. She gets home for two days and she is fine, and then she has a problem. But things are really okay.

Facilitator: It sounds very exciting, though, the prospect of being able to be back on your feet so quickly.

Catherine: Okay, so I don't have the cost of being overnight in the hospital and they didn't even, like so many doctors today, want their money up front. They said, "Just don't worry about it." It is such a loving, caring place. I'm very glad I kept the flyer. It is probably the best way for me to lose 10 pounds! *(Everyone laughs. A brief discussion about the facility ensues.)*

Note: Whenever someone raises the possibility of an operation or some medical condition, the underlying element is the *existential factor,* which often is raised by the discussion of mortality and life-threatening illnesses. The introduction of this factor often leads to other group members discussing corresponding issues.

Facilitator: Who else can check in?

Ted: I can check in. I have had them for a while. The people who know me, know I'm on medication for the hepatitis. He doesn't think there is a connection, but there are some little lumps, and I had one taken away a long time ago, and it was biopsied and there was no problem. So I showed this doctor a year ago, and he was pretty calm, but my concern was that they are in my liver area, and that's where the hepatitis is. There are lumps in here, so I am going to have minor surgery in an afternoon down at [a local hospital].

And I feel kind of like you do *(directed toward Catherine)*. I've been through a lot of things, and I'm not too fearful right now. I've got some medical things coming up. They are going to reassess my medicine. They are going to start taking me down if I stay in remission. I hope I can. The doctors here want me to go to [a large teaching hospital in the area]. I'm going to go the first week in February to have [this, this, and this] done.

My attitude has been pretty good. My numbers have been good. I'm looking forward to seeing where this is going. I want to see if this is going down or up. I want to see if there are side effects to the medicine. They don't have long-term research on this, so they don't know the side effects. They really don't know the long-term effects of the antifuron. I know some of the side effects I have right now, and I don't know what the long-term effect is.

And I was able to share with Valerie [a group member] about my daughter. She helped me last night with my daughter having a pretty bad time. We talked about the daughter and that was okay, pretty positive, but what else came in the back door was with my wife. There is another part, as people have been talking about today.

Over time I feel I have been more on a mission from God in my life, and I have been very comfortable with it. And over the years I've been getting closer, and as I've gotten closer, there is some guilt that has come up for things I had done. My wife and I had an abortion six years ago, and so I think some of this is coming from the daughter. I'm not sure where it is coming from, but it hurts. It hurts. And I don't feel good about that.

And if I think back to when I was 20 with the girlfriend in Texas, I start thinking, I killed two babies. Then, intellectually, I can tell you that was then, and I'm working through that, but sometimes I go right through that and I'm not feeling good.

So I shared that with Valerie and that was very helpful. I really did move through that. I really was feeling some guilt with my wife. I know she is having a real rough time with this stuff, too, and I can't bring that back. I can't change that. And then I am not happy with that decision. I wholeheartedly believe that, if I had it to do over, I wouldn't do that. I believe that in my heart. There has been some stuff there.

Note: It is interesting to note that the introduction of the existential factor has led to information about death. In this case the presentation about the medical condition gave way to the information about the abortion. In turn, this information led to a concern about feeling separated from a loved one. Isolation and the feeling of separateness is often the underlying focus of existential factors.

Facilitator: Uh-huh.

Ted: I'm not angry. That's how I used to handle those sort of things. I'd use the anger emotion and power through it. I'm glad I'm not doing that. That's growth for me. I used to handle it in a lot of inappropriate ways. And I'm just noticing it an awful, awful lot. I'm looking at the little kids, and I'm missing some things. They are in the pool playing. My heart is very drawn to that. There is a good side to all of this. I know it's going to come out. My wife and I have talked about adopting. Foster things. I know that we're moving. I just think that there are a lot of emotions coming up, and that's just where I'm at today.

Today was better than last night. I knew I was thinking about it. I woke up at five o'clock in the morning, BOINK! It was right there. But there was a movement from where I was at last night. I was swimming yesterday, and I see all the kids swimming and doing their lessons, so I'm going to follow through like I said. I'm definitely not going to change my plans.

In March I'll go up to New England and try to make contact and see how that goes. I feel good about that. I'm a little scared about that. I don't know which way it will go but I want to do the right thing for me and for her. So, er, it's positive. I'm scared, but I feel it's positive.

Facilitator: Sounds like there's a lot of different components to this now.

Ted: More than I realized. More than I realized. And I'm real thankful I'm here for my wife because I know she's having a hard time with this herself. I feel I wasn't straightforward when we made the decision. I don't think it was done intentionally, I just said, "I'm not sure what should we do."

Maybe I should tell you the other piece, just to add. We decided we weren't going to have children. I'm 45, she's about 38, no 40. She was fearful about having children because of my drug history. She's a nurse, and I understood that, and she was also unsure about my sobriety. But I guess in the eight or ten years she became more comfortable that I was going to stay sober and wanted to raise a child, but she still feared the drugs and we talked about some options.

She could no longer use the contraceptives that she was using. She was on the pill for many years and her system wasn't really doing well with the other one. So, I had a vasectomy. They told me everything was fine, and it was the doctor's fault, whatever you want to say, but after I had my vasectomy, she got pregnant, which really threw us a curve until we figured out what happened. They said I was at zero, but I wasn't at zero. Apparently some men have another part of whatever it is. I'm not a doctor or anything, but evidently it was letting the sperm come through and was not clipped, or whatever they do.

So she got pregnant, and we weren't sure what we were going to do. And I came in and took the play and helped make the decision about that. That didn't help. It complicated it that much more. But she's working through it.

She's got real good support from her family. Some members of her family are upset with this. She is there as much for me as I am for her. So we're glad we're talking about it. We had a child stay with us. We helped him out, and we're glad we could do that. It's not the same but I feel good about that. It's something that will make our hearts feel better. I'm trying to hold on to that.

Valerie: I just, the other day, I realized all I've been through, my kids leaving. It's such a big change. It's hard to put into words. Not bad—different, just different. It sort of reminds me when I got divorced, in a way, because I had a certain life for 12 years and then I didn't, you know, and then I didn't. It feels like the same kind of process in a way. It was different, it took time. Suddenly I realized, I'm the only one who lives here! *(Everyone laughs.)* It's not bad; it's just different. There are all these decisions to make. I make sure I invite the kids over for dinner. It was very nice. I feel so much clearer with Tommy. That feels really good. I don't feel guilty. I really have the sense he's doing what he needs to do.

Facilitator: Yeah, good.

Valerie: So that's good. My daughter, I'm surprised she came over on Monday. And when she came over I was in the middle of four things, as I usually am. I was making dinner, putting up the Christmas tree, I have to fill out forms for her, and I have to go to the store. So I said, "Hey, Suzanne, how about if you help me out?" My daughter is 18. "Do something, one of these things."

She's like, "No I don't want to do anything." She's acting like she's a guest in the house, and I'm like, "You're really not a guest here, you're my family."

And she said, "Well, you're the one who wanted a divorce. And we're not a family." She said, "You're the one who wanted a divorce." I couldn't believe it. I was like, whoa, and it put me so off because I was in the middle of all this, like, emotional pressure to get this stuff done. It's getting late.

I just said, "What are you talking about?" And those words are her father's words. That is what he always said to me when I had any problem along the way. "Well you're the one who wanted a divorce." Oh, God, when am I going to get a break here? When am I not going to be guilty for getting a divorce?

Facilitator: Yeah.

Valerie: I said, "Suzanne. I'm sorry. I just couldn't do it any longer. I'm sorry." And I said to her, "You know, we both had a choice. You had a choice, and you had an abortion. And I had a choice, and I had the baby and got married. We both had our choices here." And I said, "I'm sorry. I wouldn't have done it. I wouldn't have married your father if ... " And then afterward I said, "Oh, God, what did I say? I hope that wasn't ... " I don't know what so we dropped it. I found myself to be too defensive though, you know.

And the next day I was able to settle myself down a bit, and I said, "I'm really sorry for ... Just give me time to explain myself. I'm just, I'm just sorry that you're hurting about it." That was better for me. I didn't like the other piece of having to have her understand. She doesn't have to understand whatever my life is and was. But we did talk a little bit.

I don't know if I told you, Suzanne went away to Aruba over Christmas. And she was with a family, a Jewish family, who have plenty of money, and she's best friends with the daughter and she's been for years. And they asked her last year and she wasn't able to go. This year it was much more affordable, so she went. My poor daughter was traumatized because, every day, all they did was argue. Did I tell you that? I think I might have told you *(to Ted)*.

Don: All they did was what?

Valerie: Argue. Constantly. All they did was argue. All they did was argue. Suzanne came back a wreck. This was too much. Everyday for nine days. Everyday since she came off the plane, she got off the plane and called me: "I couldn't take it." I felt bad for not being able to tell these people that, because they ... I can't call them and say thank you for taking my daughter, because I don't feel like that right now. Suzanne came back after all that saying, "I may not have their money, but I am happy." She came back with some good stuff, but I am sorry she had to go through all of that. But I said to her, "If I had stayed married to your father, that's what it would have been."

Facilitator: That's what would have been there.

Valerie: "That's *exactly* what would have happened. We were arguing all the time. I wouldn't have wished that for you." She didn't have to live through that. So she didn't live through that.

So when she said, "We are not a family," I said, "There are all types of families, they come in all types of shapes and forms. They don't have to be mother, father, and two kids." I felt very strongly. I said, "If you don't want to be a family, that is your choice. As far as I'm concerned, we're a family."

But I think that she is going through her own stuff again about the divorce. She's been with her father a couple of months, and I guess other parts are coming up. And it was fine after we talked.

This is her own process, other than taking my own responsibility. And so that was that. I called her and she apologized to me. I can't take on guilt with this. I did the best I could. I don't know what else to do with it. I did talk to my son about it. I told him that Suzanne seems upset about the divorce, and he said, "It's fine with me." That's my son. The only thing with that was that it was financially very hard.

Note: The group theme that seems to be emerging from the initial check-in until now is the feeling of being separated from family. It appears to have evolved, at least partially, along the lines of existential factors. People in the group are sharing about their alienation and separation. You will notice that even when Melanie shared, she was a *polarity* for the group. She was talking about how good she felt when she had developed a coping mechanism, a sense of relief from her anger and separateness from her father. A fairly strong theme is building.

Don: Whew, boy, all that stuff is bringing up, I mean, from every part.

Facilitator: Yeah. We covered the field today.

Don: We started off talking about the death at the opera thing. [A major figure from the opera world died on stage just as he was singing, "No one ever lives forever." Don was in the audience in a very good seat, from which he saw the man fall 30 feet after suffering a heart attack.] Talking about illness and cancer, I have been trying to make some decisions for myself, too, because with the history I have with my father dying of colon cancer, I am supposedly a prime candidate. I'm supposed to be careful what I eat and have a big fiber diet. About two years after my father died, I had some bleeding, and I went to the doctor, and I had some tests and a barium, and he said, "There are some less serious things that are causing this that we can deal with." But he still wanted me to be checked.

When I left my profession [the priesthood], I was no longer entitled to very elaborate health care examinations. So finally, last January, I went because I was a little concerned. I went to see a gastroenterologist, and he examined me, and he said, "I think it's a good idea. I would like to do a colonoscopy." I was still covered by health insurance, which was a good thing because it turned out to be—for an in-out thing—it turned out to be three thousand dollars. But that's because they found polyps.

It was so scary. I was still on the table waking up, and the doctor is handing me photographs, *photographs*! "Here's what we found in your colon." Shows me the polyp and the biopsy. So that's why, when I went back, he said, "Basically with this type of thing there's two types of tissue. The type that is dying and the other type that, if left alone, will become malignant, and this is the kind that will become malignant." I want you to come in next year.

Anyway, to make a long story short, here were things that happened with the doctor that made me lose respect for the doctor. I didn't like how I was treated. Something went wrong with my arm. I don't know if they had the IV wrong. My whole arm was purple, yellow, and green, and it hurt for weeks. The doctor made like this was nothing. When I called the office they told me to go see my GP, that I didn't have to see a gastroenterologist about a bruised arm. And I said, "Yeah, but this happened in your office. Aren't you concerned about that?" So anyway, I didn't go back this year, and I've been thinking about it and wondering about those people who told me that three years is frequent enough to have a colonoscopy. So I've been trying to decide about that. And my mother has bleeding, and she went for some tests and she has to go for more. She has a history of bladder infections, so they don't think that it is anything more than that, but they don't know. And after this thing that happened at the opera ...

Facilitator: What a night at the opera!

Note: The existential theme and the sense that we are, indeed, alone in this world are now firmly established in the group. It is interesting to note that the real time that has elapsed is not more than a half hour, and yet a strong theme of death and isolation has been established.

Don: Now I am thinking about death all of a sudden, which is not something that I've done for a long, long time. It was 10 years ago that my father was terminally ill and I was thinking about Pat and me. And I even called him up one night and talked about how dying is not something you do with someone. You do it by yourself. One of us is going to go and leave the other one behind. And I didn't know where it was coming from. It was pretty horrendous. But I talked to people about it, and I know that always helps. I am coming out of that panicky anxiety feeling and getting some spiritual peace, which follows the holidays.

And I guess I am wrestling with the health insurance thing, because I know I am covered until the end of May—but beyond that I don't know. But there are a couple of good things in the air. First of all, here is somebody that doesn't have health insurance and she *(to Catherine)* is handling it! And then you *(to Valerie)* said something that was very comforting, but I forgot what it was. Tomorrow I'm going up to see Pat's therapist. We went once before the holidays, and I just feel that this is something that I would like to do, because this time I have somebody who is not afraid to talk and work things out. So I believe I would really benefit by taking advantage of that. What's happening is that the last relationship I was in was such a struggle constantly and so dramatic, and it was really all about me not accepting the person for who he was.

Facilitator: Uh, hm.

Don: He was never going to change no matter what I was going to do. I was trying to make him be somebody else. Nevertheless, every little thing, I've been noticing, that comes up between Pat and me starts, if I am not real careful, starts dragging me back into the old pattern again. As before, the message to myself was: You shouldn't feel that way. You are so needy and making excuses, trying to paint a rosy picture. When I should be telling myself: This relationship isn't really for you. You have been taking a lot of emotional abuse. And now the tables are turned and now the messages are trying to pull me away and turning Pat into the bad guy, so to speak. This is the time when I should be saying: No, this is my issue that is coming up. This has nothing to do with him. But it's not working. It's working in reverse. So I want to go in tomorrow and talk about this [with Pat's therapist].

And the last thing just happened: I stopped at my mother's for lunch to leave my pet bird with her for the weekend. When I'm sitting with my mother talking, she gets this glassed-over look like she is tuning out or whatever, and then I'll feel like an insinuation of a tear, and I have no idea what's going on. And she, like, doesn't want to talk about it, and it turns out—today it finally came out—and it turned my stomach and I was so mad at my mother.

I finally, last summer, with Pat, I wrote my brother a letter, because I was getting nowhere. They are very strange down there. They have a pay phone. They don't answer their phone. They don't return calls. I wrote him on some birthday cards, "Please call me some night. I would really like to talk to you about a few things."

A few years ago when he was in mid-life crisis and trauma, he called me all distraught over the stuff that happened in our childhood, but now he doesn't want to talk to me. So I wrote him this letter saying I appreciated how I felt I may have hurt him, how he hurt me, and what I appreciate about him. Along with it, I also thought that it was about time I told him that I was gay. He was the only family member that didn't know. So along with that, I also explained a few changes in my life that were changing about my parents, how I learned to see my mother and father differently and forgive my father, all the while acknowledging that he was a rage-aholic and there were a lot of things that shouldn't have been the way they were. And my mother, after my father died, I had become, like, her surrogate husband, which wasn't helping. And I had to detach from that and recognize it for what it was and deal with it. So I am telling you [his brother] all this to help you understand where I am at in my life right now.

He was so enraged that letter would say these things about my mother and father, or maybe he was angry about the me-being-gay part, being a priest, or how it came out, I don't know. I have no idea because there is no communication. He told my mother this! Everything that was in the letter. This is what her tears were about. I just couldn't believe it.

And then it hit home to me again, it was the same old story. I should have known better. I should have accepted my brother for who he is. He is this 4-year-old little boy walking around in an adult body. That no matter what kind of tragedy that happens in somebody else's life, he makes it about him. Suddenly it becomes all about him. "Poor me." And he doesn't care who. I couldn't believe he said those things to my mother. What purpose could he have had? So I had a talk with her, and I did explain myself, and she seemed—I guess enough time has passed that she seemed—less hurt. I tried to put things into perspective for her. There were a few things I didn't say that he quoted and twisted around. Anyway.

So the ride down here was a spiritual getting back on track. Recognizing my anger and then letting go of it. Not jumping back into my old self—which would be to right away do something about it, to jump out of the car, write this nasty letter, and stick it in the mailbox now. Or cancel my trip for the weekend, or call him and blast him on the phone—none of which is going to help me.

Facilitator: Although we could do it here. (*Everyone laughs.*)

Note: This is the beginning of the *enactment stage*. We are warmed up to the action. Don is very much with his feelings, and the group is clearly involved with the theme. You will notice that each person in the group has had a chance to share, and now Don. He is perhaps the most animated about his condition, and it pulled together the central issues being presented by all members. Both

Don and Valerie had issues that were current and ongoing in their lives and that pertained to the central theme.

Don: Yes. *(Laughing.)*

Facilitator: Would you want to do that? Would you be willing to do that?

Don: I don't *want* to. *(Laughing.)*

Facilitator: I changed it right away. I knew.

Don: I know better. I've been doing this stuff long enough. I don't want to. No. But, yes, I am willing to.

Note: It is better not to ask the protagonist if he or she "wants" to do a drama. It is most likely that he or she does not really *want* to do one, but he or she might be willing to proceed.

Facilitator: Can you pick somebody to be him?

Don: Holy mackerel. *(Everyone laughs.)* It's hard to pick somebody.

Facilitator: We can use an empty chair if you like.

Note: See Chapter 2 for a full description of using the *empty chair*. The choice in this instance reflects the fact that Don would rather not have members of the group serve as an *auxiliary* as his brother. This is perfectly acceptable and allows for a *monodrama* to take place. In these instances, when the protagonist has chosen not to have an auxiliary, there are a few guidelines to keep in mind:

1. When using the empty chair, it is important to have the protagonist reverse roles with the person in the vacant seat. This process allows the protagonist to become aware of the perspective of the other person and, in doing so, develop either a strategy for coping with this person or new ways of viewing the situation.

2. After protagonists have reversed roles with the empty chair, they must return to their own roles. This completes the process of *role reversal.*

3. Quite often the outcome for the protagonist of such an intense piece of work is a catharsis of some sort.

Don: I really have a hard time picking any of these nice people here to play . . .

Facilitator: . . . to play the brother from hell. How far apart should these be? *(Don chooses an empty chair on the far side of the room to play his brother. Other group members laugh at the distance he chooses.)*

Why don't you reverse roles, start over there *(in the empty chair)* as your brother. *(Don goes across the room to the other chair and sits down.)*

(to Don who is playing his brother) What is your name?

Don: *(as his brother)* John.

Facilitator: And how old are you, John?

Don: *(as his brother)* Forty-six.

Facilitator: And can you tell us a little bit about your brother, Don?

Don: *(to the facilitator)* You mean about the incident? Or in general?

Facilitator: In general.

Don: In general. *(Continues, as his brother.)* When we were growing up, my brother was a real sissy and a mama's boy. He hung around with weird friends and everything. He was always playing weird games in the house. Mom and Dad always stuck up for him. I got blamed for everything.

Facilitator: How many years apart are you?

Don: *(as his brother)* Three years apart. And then when he got to high school, it seemed like he had everything, and I had nothing. He was so talented and all this music and everything. No matter what he did, it was great. Everybody loved it. No matter what I did, I got in trouble. I was depressed, and I couldn't finish anything. Didn't finish high school. I put Mom and Dad through a lot. I wanted to kill myself. They took me to psychiatrists, and I got thrown out of Catholic school.

Facilitator: So you didn't like him very much.

Don: *(as his brother)* I think I liked him, but he was just a threat to me. I would rather not deal with him and go my own way and let him go his way. That's all.

Facilitator: Okay. Now reverse roles. *(Don gets up, crosses the room, and sits back in his original chair.)*

How does this encounter begin?

Don: I guess I'd like to know why none of my notes and phone calls were responded to and why you weren't willing to talk to me when I asked you and told you I had some things about my childhood that I wanted to talk to you about.

Note: Often the best time to have the protagonist reverse roles is after a question has been asked.

Facilitator: Reverse roles. *(Don changes chairs.)*

Don: *(as his brother)* I don't have time for that stuff. You wouldn't know what it's like. I have a family and bills to pay, and my wife and I were arguing about the money for our son to go to college. I didn't want him to go to New York City to go to this thing, and she thought it was a good idea. You know I had that accident with my knee—I don't even know if you know about that—when I was coaching that baseball team. And I was in so much pain, going to therapy, and nobody even called me.

Facilitator: Reverse roles. *(Don changes chairs.)*

Don: I don't think it has anything to do with your knee. Nothing has changed. It has always been this way. Mom has been telling us she can't get through to you. You have the tape machine on and you don't call back. She never knows when she is going to hear from you. And when you were upset years ago on Christmas, you call me up all in tears and everything about your crisis. All I wanted to do is talk to you, and you can't be bothered. I think the stuff about your knee is important, too. I didn't know about it until the Monday after it happened. You never called to tell me you were hurt. How was I supposed to know?

Facilitator: Reverse roles. *(Don changes chairs).*

Don: *(as his brother)* Oh, that's bullshit. I told Mom I can't be spending a bunch of money calling people up in Colorado and you in New Jersey. I'm sure she told you. Don't give me that excuse.

Facilitator: Reverse roles. *(Don shakes his head as he walks back to his chair and makes a circular motion with his right index finger to indicate the futility of the conversation.)* Right, and on it goes. So let's bring it to the current issue.

Don: That was a really lousy thing you did, telling Mom all the details of what's going on in my life. Pouring my heart out to you, and you going back and telling Mom. I don't know what you could possibly hope to accomplish by that. That was a really lousy thing you did last summer when, after you got the letter, you responded by telling me I was no longer the legal guardian of your children. Asking me for a copy of the will back, sending me two dollars for postage. Why would I want to talk to you now.

Facilitator: Reverse roles. *(Don gets up and changes chairs.)*

Don: *(as his brother)* Well, it didn't have anything to do with that. George was turning 18, and he could be his own guardian and Gregory's guardian. It was just a coincidence it happened then. It doesn't have anything to do with it.

Facilitator: Will you now just stand behind the chair and be his double. What's he really feeling toward you?

Note: The facilitator has a choice of using the protagonist or other members in the group to double the feelings of the protagonist. Considering the nature of the drama at this point, a decision was made by the facilitator to declare this a monodrama and to allow the protagonist the opportunity to play all the roles available.

Don: *(as his brother's double)* I think he felt angry and disappointed because I was always the one holding the golden torch, and it was very ... I think he was blaming me because he knew that my mother was feeling let down by my leaving the priesthood. And like I said, he has always made everything about himself. And the fact that, on top of everything else, I have a brother who is gay. Now I have to deal with that.

Facilitator: Reverse roles back to your position. *(Don does this.)* Stand behind the chair [thus becoming his own double]. And can you express some of your anger toward him?

Note: The use of the double in this instance has allowed the protagonist, while in the role of his brother's double and his own, to feel the depth of the pain of separation and distance and sadness. The purpose of doing this is to allow for the expression of the deeper, not fully expressed emotions to be vented. The opportunity for a catharsis at this point is very good.

Don: *(Long pause, then he starts to cry)* You really make me feel shitty. You were supposed to be my big brother. You were never there for me when I was little. You mock me, make fun of me in front of my own friends. Then I reach out to you to tell you who I really am and you respond by going away. We had to do everything with Mom by ourselves *(crying and voice raised)*. When Dad was dying, you didn't come until the last weekend, when Mom begged you to come so you could see him while he was alive *(now yelling)*. And you spent the whole weekend fixing doorknobs and going to AA meetings. You couldn't even go in the room and be with him. And you didn't bring your kids up to see Mom for 10 years since Dad died. Now you're blaming me for saying something to Mom about Dad that's true. You haven't been a part of this family since you moved to Florida. So don't try to tell me what I should be doing. You don't want to be part of this family, *FINE*. Stay in Florida. I don't care if I ever talk to you again. Stay there and be alone. We don't need you.

Facilitator: Can you say the last thing you want to say to him for right now?

Note: This allows for some degree of closure to take place for the protagonist and begins the reentry back into the group.

Don:	*(As his own double still—he is much more composed than a few moments ago, but still sobbing.)* I have reached out to you for the last time. I say it is all up to you now *(breathing very deeply and crying, takes a long pause).* I started talking about this with my mother when it came out. She said, "Your father died at the right time. He missed all the fun in the last couple of years *(long pause— he is still sobbing).* It just seems like I am the one who was supposed to be perfect, and now that I am not, I am ruining everybody's life in the family.
Facilitator:	Um-hum.
Don:	It's too bad. It's too bad. They have to make their own life and plan their own happiness. It's not up to me to do it for them *(a brief pause, then a sigh of relief).* Whew.
Facilitator:	As you get ready, let's come back to the group and see where people are at with that. *(Don sits back down in the group, and the chairs are pulled back into the circle.)*
	(talking to Don) So, Don, I am going to ask people to share with you what kind of things came up for them. Don't feel obligated to respond. Just take it in.

Note: The group now begins to share their thoughts and feelings to Don's psychodrama. This signals the beginning of the *sharing stage* and continues the healing process.

Catherine:	It just seems like such a game in the family. And you tried to be so honest to everyone—and that was painful

Don: Nobody wants to talk about it.

Facilitator: So what kinds of things did people get in touch with as they watched Don do this.

Ted: I don't have a good relationship with my brother. I don't know if I can keep reaching out and reaching out. And the door just shuts. I keep wanting to reach out and make another attempt. Part of me wants to do it, and another part of me doesn't want to do it, because I don't feel the acknowledgment from him. Certainly the frustration was coming up as I watched this. I keep telling myself he is sick.

My mom has a lot of conflict with my brother, and I tell her she has to deal with it her way. That I have my way of dealing with it. That I can't tell her. What struck me the most was that I can't reach out much more. It is taking too much out of me. I go through so much after. I hear a call on the tape machine, and part of me wants to return it, and part of me doesn't. Nothing has really changed in the last 8 to 10 years in terms of me wanting to reach out. There are two years difference between me and my brother. In terms of age we could pal around, but that's about it.

Melanie: When I was listening to you, there were two words that I found: "betrayal" and "humiliation." And I can just picture it. My dad used to do that to me in front of my family. If I wasn't home in time to get dinner started or to have dinner, he would start to whistle for me like I was a dog. One time he came down the street to get me, and he started kicking me to get back home with my friends standing around looking. I just blocked out whatever happened so I would be able to face him again. I don't have any siblings, but my two kids are 12 months apart, and that really hurts me. But they are going to have to handle whatever goes on between them.

Catherine: Your brother's part is interesting to me. I think the only way you could have a relationship with him is if you talk about him. But it doesn't work if you have to talk about you.

Note: During this sharing, people are directing their comments back to Don. Often the depth of the sharing allows for a secondary protagonist to emerge with his or her own issues. When this happens, a "spin-off" psychodrama may take place. It is a continuation of the work begun by the first protagonist.

We will return to this group and its spin-off drama after the next chapter on sociometry, transference, and tele.

Chapter 5

SOCIOMETRY, TRANSFERENCE, AND TELE

The core therapeutic group process is interaction between members, and action methods enhance interaction. The organizing principle behind interactive techniques is *sociometry*. Sociometry is the measure of the strength of attraction or repulsion between people based on different criteria. It appears that connecting with other people is an inherent impulse. We are drawn to relate to each other. However, the manner in which our connectedness has evolved and the history of our relationships with other people can make connections threatening and dangerous as well as delightful and desirable. The goal of group psychotherapy is to make connections safer and the motivation behind interactions understood.

Sociometry shows how we connect to different people based on different criteria. If you were asked, "Who would you borrow ten dollars from?" you would most likely give a very different answer from the one you'd give if you were asked, "What person irritates you the most?" As a facilitator, when you change the question, you change the criteria, and in changing the criteria, you change the way people connect to one another. When this happens, you have altered the sociometry. People hooked up together at one level may be unhooked at another level. Asking participants with whom they would have liked to play as a child probably would yield a different answer than asking with whom they would want to write an academic paper. Sociometry is the fabric of the connections in a group. Understanding sociometry is a bit like understanding why different crops grow better in different climates, in different soils, and under different conditions. If you change the conditions, crops that could not grow before will flourish, while the usual harvest will diminish.

> **Case of Edith.** Edith, a depressed woman with very low status in the group due to her severe withdrawal, had an uncanny ability for interpreting dreams. Once the members in the group realized this ability, they would bring their dreams to the group with the request that Edith give her interpretation of the symbolism. She had not been chosen for actions by other members before this ability was recognized. After her strength was revealed, the criteria changed, and she became a much more integrated and valued member of the group.

SOCIOMETRIC CHOICES

The law of *sociodynamic energy* says, simply, that all our choices and preferences are not equal. This seems so obvious it is hardly worth mentioning, yet it is the very fiber behind group dynamics, indeed, the fiber behind the conditions in our life. Who we choose to spend our time with, who we avoid, who we are drawn to but inhibit ourselves from being with, and who we are repelled by but fail to avoid all determine the interactions in our lives. Consider a group of six of your associates that you work with or go to school with. If I asked you to rank them in terms of who you would want to have lunch with, you probably could narrow your choice down to one or two people from the group. You will be willing to spend more energy on one person than on others. Your choices are not equal. Sociometry measures the strength of these choices. It measures the variability of the sociodynamic energy between people.

Given this variability, the strength of your attraction toward others and theirs toward you are not always equal. You might choose someone to have lunch with and he or she might choose you as well. This would be a *reciprocal choice,* indicating that you are mutually attracted to each other. But what happens if you choose someone and he or she chooses someone other than you? Or, if someone chooses you who is not the person you are choosing?

The group psychotherapy situation enables us to realize these attractions, repulsions, and indifferences while we experiment with new ways of interacting and communicating with others. Action methods offer a chance to demonstrate these choices in a manner that invites exploration. One of the strong benefits of using action techniques is their graphic nature. Rather than guessing at what people are thinking or inferring it from their words or interactions, you can ask them to *show* you what they are thinking and feeling. This cuts down on guessing, and makes private reactions public.

Large movement techniques (action methods designed for participation by a large number of people) are designed to help people get warmed up to the process of interacting and self-disclosing to one another. The nonthreatening nature of these interactions allows group members to become ready to be with one another and to reveal their thoughts and feelings.

Once you move to exercises that involve sociometric choices, such as choosing a double or an auxiliary (see Chapter 2), you raise the emotional ante for the group. Members make choices based on who they are drawn to and who they are less drawn to. The issue of choice is placed directly in front of each person. They are confronted with the questions: "Who will I choose? Who will I leave out? Who is choosing me? Who has not chosen me? Why have I made my choices? Why have they made theirs?" All of these questions really tug at the threads of our awareness. They beg to be answered, explored, or at least acknowledged. Noticing sociometric choices in action moves people into an encounter with others as well as with themselves. These questions allow us to examine transference and tele.

TRANSFERENCE AND TELE

Transference is a concept Freud advanced early in his theory of psychoanalysis. In brief, the concept involves the transfer of feelings from one person to another. Feelings developed earlier for other people (usually parents) are later transferred to others. Transference is a one-way distortion that obscures one's perception. Group therapy offers the potential for multiple transferences as well as an enhanced opportunity to explore them. Exploration of transferences is a primary task of the group. Members learn to recognize when transferential feelings are activated and acquire coping strategies that lead to healthier interactions among members. Ultimately the learning that takes place in the group evolves to the point that it is applied to relationships outside of the group.

While Freud's contribution to understanding the psyche was enormous, there were several glaring holes in his theory. Most notable was the lack of even an acknowledgment that a spontaneous interaction takes place between people. However, Moreno (1951) has provided us with the concept of *tele*. Tele is, simply, the feeling that surrounds an interaction between people. It is the natural, unfiltered experience that takes place when people encounter each other. The "chemistry" or the "vibes" you get from interactions with others, or the impression you have of how they would be to interact with, is tele. While transference is one-directional and pathological in nature, tele is a reciprocal and natural process.

If I see someone who reminds me of my mother (she talks, sits, acts, or does something that reminds me of my mother), I can have a positive, negative, or split transference. I might have a positive reaction to this woman because she reminds me of the positive aspects of my mother. Or I might have a negative reaction if the unpleasant features of my mother are enacted. I would have a split transference if I were aware that the woman had neither all good or all bad aspects of my mother, but some of both.

Split transference is as close as Freud gets to acknowledging the fact that, in interactions with others, the real aspects of the person onto whom the transference is projected can weaken the transference. You might have a negative transference toward someone but find aspects of his or her behavior tolerable or even noble.

The concept of tele describes the real or natural interaction that takes place between people. Further, this natural reaction is reciprocal. However, the reciprocal process does not have to be complementary or symmetrical. For example, I might have a positive telic reaction to someone who has a neutral telic reaction to me. There are three types of general reactions that you can have toward a person: positive, negative, and neutral. In turn, others may have these three reactions toward you. These reactions can occur at initial encounters and may change over time as you get to know a person. Telic reactions are free of transferences. They are your natural feelings with a person. While tele is two-way, nonpathological, and continually being re-assessed and reevaluated, transference is one-way, pathological (due to the distorted projection), and a relatively fixed reaction. When you add positive, negative, and neutral telic reactions to the positive, negative, and split transferential possibilities, you can sense just how much is going on when two people encounter each other!

Consider the following encounter. You have a positive attraction to a man based on his looks and his manners. As you spend time with him, you notice that he has a rather short fuse and the way in which he displays his temper is very uncomfortable, yet familiar to you. He seems indifferent to you; you sense neither a positive nor a negative reaction to you. The question in this encounter is: How much of your reactions toward each other is based on transferences and how much is based on tele?

SOCIOMETRIC ROLE POSITIONS

Four sociometric role positions may be occupied within a group. Each position reflects a different choice members make with each other. The choices are based on specific responses that have manifested in the group but have not been validated by specific questioning. The four positions are: sociometric star, star of incongruity, negative star, and isolate.

A star is a person who has been chosen by the group to represent the group on a particular issue. The key word in this sentence is "chosen." The sociometric star is a positive choice. People see the issue this person represents or the manner of his or her presentation as something they can relate to, something they can learn from. They choose the star based on a question asked by the facilitator. There is a desire, or at least a tolerance, to be the star. Choosing the star position is a positive interaction, a choice made by several toward one. In the group, when a question is asked, people are told to put their hands on the shoulder of the person they are choosing. In this way, the choice is graphic and personal. As the facilitator you can see how the energy in the group is formed. The person with the most choices would be the sociometric star. People with two or more choices are stars, but the person with the most choices is *the* star. There are eight conditions under which a person is chosen or not chosen:

Positive Star (Sociometric Star)

1. When you want to be chosen (or it is okay that you are chosen) and people choose you.

   In this condition, there is positive energy because of the mutual reciprocity. If the individual chosen has reservations about being chosen or is unable to accept the feedback, he or she is an ambivalent star.

Ambivalent Star (Star of Incongruity)

2. When you are indifferent to the choice and are chosen.

3. When you don't want to be chosen and you are chosen.

   These two positions create the star of incongruity or ambivalence. If you do not change your feeling after you are chosen, you are likely to sabotage yourself as a way of getting out of the role. This is often the underlying reason behind self-defeating or self-destructive behaviors. When people are placed in roles they do not want to be in, they will try to get themselves out of the role.

Rejection Star (Negative Star)

4. When you want to be chosen and are not.

5. When you are indifferent to being chosen and are not.

6. When you are chosen (but wish not to be) because you display undesirable characteristics perceived by others.

7. When you are chosen (and wish to be) because you display undesirable characteristics perceived by others.

These conditions form rejection or negative stars. There is a great deal of energy in being chosen as a rejection star. In the group, if you asked, "Who is the person you feel most inhibited by?" the person with the most choices would be a rejection star. Making covert feelings known through a sociometric choice provides graphic feedback for the individual. Once you have made this information available, he or she then may be able to assimilate it in such a way as to help change his or her interpersonal manner.

Isolate

8. When you do not want to choose or be chosen and are not.

This is the isolate position. Moreno (1951, 1956, 1978) referred to a person who is continually in this position as an "organic" isolate, neither choosing nor being chosen. Typically, the way to change the position of the isolate is to have him or her identify to the group how he or she feels in the position. Once he or she has been able to do this, others can relate to him or her, and this changes how people fee toward the isolate. If individuals are able to identify the feelings behind their isolation, others may be able to relate to them more readily.

With this understanding of sociometry, transference, and tele, let's return to the transcript of the group to follow the drama that takes place.

Chapter 6

ACTION METHODS IN USE: CONTINUED FROM CHAPTER 4

As you will recall, as Chapter 4 ended, Don had just completed his drama and the group was making their comments as part of the sharing. Each person was noting how the drama affected him or her and was relating feedback to Don. We pick up where Valerie was sharing her reactions.

Valerie: My mother called to tell me that my brother stole money from her. I wanted to get off the phone with her and kill him. I felt like you. I waited another few days, because I knew he was trying to talk to her about her finances. I am glad I didn't get in the middle of it. I don't want to do it. I don't want to get in the middle of it. I don't want to talk about his negative stuff. I don't want to do this anymore.

Betsy: I kept thinking about my old family. I mean my mom and dad and my sister and myself. We never really talk about anything. I mean, you know, my mom talks about whatever she is feeling is going on with my father, and that's about it. She used to try to pull me in, but that I stopped. My sister would do things that would really upset my mom, and I would tell mom to let it go, then she saw that I wouldn't really play along with it. The only thing is that my sister will get me on the phone and tell me all the things she does for my mother and her daughter. I don't ever say anything, because she isn't the one that does anything. But anything she does, if she buys them anything, she's a compulsive buyer, I guess she tries to lay a guilt trip on me about it. There again, those things don't both me either, because my feelings are, she doesn't have anything else to do. But every now and then I would like to say those things, like, "Hey, you don't have anything else to do!" But I don't. I keep everything inside.

Facilitator: Well, we have time now. *(Everyone laughs.)* Would you be willing to say some of these things?

Note: This is an invitation for Betsy to continue the session by engaging in her own psychodrama. This is the beginning of a spin-off.

Betsy: You know, I can say it. I thought about it the other day while I was driving the car. I always hear, "How good your sister is. How good your sister is. She always is doing this for that one or doing this for this one." She buys. It's not her money. She doesn't work.

Facilitator: Right.

Betsy: She doesn't do anything but shop. *(Everybody laughs.)* Talk about dysfunction. Nobody ever talks about all the people she has hurt. She's hurt an awful lot of people in one lifetime. And I think about all the things, even for myself, that she's done.

When I got a divorce, my mind was gone. Everything was all a mess. So I asked her and her husband if they would store things for me. She just let her kids get at it. She let her kids totally destroy pictures that had sentimental value. They just totally destroyed it. She never said she was sorry it happened. Just nothing. I don't know how to explain it. She doesn't have any regard for other people's feelings. She'll tell you she does, but every time you talk to her ... She treats men unbelievably. The worse she treats them, the better she gets treated. There's a part of her that's as mean as can be, and then there's that other part.

Facilitator: So what is it that you wanted to say to her? Could you pick somebody to play her, or do we have the same dilemma?

Betsy: We have the same dilemma.

Facilitator: We don't want to put *that* on anybody.

Betsy: There is a part of her that is good and nice and fine. When she is in a good place, you couldn't ask for anybody nicer or funnier or whatever. To tell you the truth, I don't know what I will say.

Facilitator: Well, we have time to experiment. *(Everyone laughs.)*

Betsy: Oh.

Facilitator: Is that right? That she can be tough to talk to?

Betsy: Yeah. One thing just came up. The only time I ever said anything to her was one time. She became verbally abusive, and I told her I was not going to let her verbally abuse me. I told her when she calmed down to call me back. She did, two years later.

Facilitator: Some people are slower than others. *(Everyone is laughing.)*

Betsy: And she did apologize that time for her childishness. But it's when she tells me all the things she does for my parents. I just don't know how to respond to that. She does this for them or buys that for them.

Facilitator: Let's reverse roles. Let's just start over here and be her.

Betsy: Okay.

Facilitator: And what's your name?

Betsy: Her name?

Facilitator: Uh-huh.

Betsy: Margaret.

Facilitator: Okay. So, Margaret, could you tell Betsy all the things you are doing for your parents?

Note: This technique of reversing roles with the auxiliary prior to the drama has the advantage of keeping protagonists off balance by asking them to reflect on the situation at hand through the eyes of the auxiliary. This provides empathic awareness as well as an introduction of the auxiliary to the group.

Betsy: *(as Margaret)* I just bought Dad a new coat and it was really nice, and I took Mom shopping, and I was just over to the house.

Facilitator: Now would you reverse roles, but be your double behind the chair.

Betsy: Behind the chair?

Facilitator: Right. What are you thinking and feeling?

Betsy: What I think and feel?

Facilitator: Now she [Margaret] might not hear this because you haven't expressed it yet.

Betsy: How I feel? There is a part of me that I say to myself ... [Now Betsy is her own double saying how she thinks she is feeling in reaction to what Margaret has said.] ... when she tells me this I say, "That's nice, that's nice."

Facilitator: Yes. But it sounds like there is something else going on there.

Betsy: I don't feel guilty, but I just don't want to hear it.

Facilitator: How come?

Betsy: Because of her motivation. That's what it is. That's what it says to me. See how good I am. She does all these things.

Facilitator: What might you want to say to her about that. This conversation has never taken place, but ...

Betsy: Yeah. I guess I would say I don't want to hear it. I am uncomfortable with it. I get angry. I don't know what I feel. I think I have let it go for so long that now I don't know what I am feeling. That's how I responded for years: "That's nice. Gee, that's *really* nice." *(Everyone laughs.)*

Facilitator: Right.

Betsy: So I don't know what I feel.

Facilitator: Well, that's what we're going to try and find out. So let's experiment with a couple of different emotions that would seem relevant. Then we can see which one captures you. It sounds like anger is there, that you might be angry. Can you try an angry response? Remember, this is kind of protected because this is the double [referring to the role she is currently playing].

Betsy: *(as her double in a slightly raised voice)* I really don't need to hear this.

Betsy: *(as herself)* That's about the end of my angry response.

Facilitator: Okay. Would you be willing to experiment with turning it up half a notch? Making it more intense?

Betsy: I *really* don't need to hear this!

Facilitator: Reverse roles. *(The facilitator points to Margaret's vacant chair.)*

Betsy: She'll flip out.

Facilitator: *(As Betsy is moving to the other chair, the facilitator talks to her.)* Could you flip out for us? How would she flip out?

Betsy: She'd yell. That's what I don't like to do. I don't like to yell.

Facilitator: So, she does most of the yelling.

Betsy: I don't have to listen to it. But she ... *(now begins talking as Margaret)* Maybe you need to hear it. *(now in a somewhat louder voice)* After all ...

Facilitator: Can you turn that up a notch or two?

Betsy: MAYBE YOU NEED TO HEAR IT. I'M ALWAYS RUNNING MOM AND DAD AROUND, AND YOU NEVER HELP OUT. *(now as herself)* Only she would do it a lot louder.

Facilitator: Would you be willing to turn up the volume on this?

Betsy: The same thing?

Facilitator: Yeah.

Betsy: *(as Margaret)* I get tired of doing everything for Mom and Dad, and you're never around to help with Mom and Dad.

Facilitator: I'm just going to add a little bit to that. *(Now the facilitator enters the process as the double of Margaret for the purpose of amplification—he is nearly screaming.)* YOU'RE NEVER AROUND FOR MOM AND DAD. *(as the facilitator)* What was that like to hear and feel that?

Betsy: I don't like it. I don't like it.

Facilitator: Is that what she does?

Betsy: Yeah. The same as my father. I knew when my father would go into a rage that I was going to get it.

Note: This is a decision point for the facilitator using action methods. When Betsy brings up the fact that her feelings with her sister are similar to the feelings with her father, it may be an opportunity to explore that connection, review the transferential properties of her father-daughter relationship. Because this is spin-off drama, there isn't enough time to explore this piece of insight. This would be important for future work, but not possible now.

Facilitator: Reverse roles. Now when that side comes up, it gets a little intense. What happens to you on this side?

Betsy: *(as herself)* I am just shaking. Just shaking.

Facilitator: Can you now stand behind your chair—that's your double—and put some words to the shaking?

Betsy: I don't know what comes next. I am not afraid to physically take care of myself. I know I can, but it is the out-of-controlness. I can't handle the out-of-controlness. I have trouble with people out of control and that is out of control. So I don't know what to do with it.

Facilitator: I guess that would explain why you don't want to become angry. Because then you'd become like them.

Betsy: Yeah.

Facilitator: Then you too would be out of control. So by all means—don't get angry.

Betsy: In my first marriage, my first husband ... we got divorced. He was a quiet person, but it was all emotional. He never would raise his voice. We didn't have any of that. I gravitated toward him because he was a quiet person.

Facilitator: Right.

Betsy: I didn't have that.

Facilitator: But he acted it out in other ways.

Betsy: That's it. Then I got into *this* marriage. Oh, my God! It was going into the fire! He beats my father—not physical. But you think he's going to scream his head off. I am not afraid of it as I used to be. I don't like it.

Facilitator: Right.

Betsy: I just don't like it. I shut right off. I can't deal with anybody that is out of control. In my professional life I can. But not with others.

Facilitator: What would you need to feel safe right now? You said you were feeling a little shaky and nervous. Is there anything you could do with the group that would help?

Betsy: Just talking about it. I will settle right down. My leaving helps. *(Everyone laughs.)* But talking settles me right down.

Facilitator: So, is it all right for us to spend another moment or two with this?

Betsy: Okay.

Facilitator: Okay. It sounds to me like, when you are in this place, that it's either no feeling, that you are numb to the feeling, or it is pure anxiety.

Betsy: It's both. I think the anxiety is fear, yeah. Then no feelings. I have the feeling of anxiety, but outside of that I don't have anything. I close down. I grew up in a home situation where I learned to cut off from my feelings.

Facilitator: I am going to ask you to reverse roles with her [Margaret], and would you tell me what allows you to lose it from time to time? What allows you to lose it from time to time?

Betsy: *(as Margaret)* No consequences.

Facilitator: No consequences.

Betsy: *(as Margaret)* None, ever, ever. No matter what I do there is never any consequences.

Facilitator: Uh-huh. So you can raise your voice, you can be angry, and no matter what you do there is no . . .

Betsy: *(as Margaret)* Nothing. There is nothing ever. There's no consequences. As a kid growing up, in my marriage, nothing.

Facilitator: Could you show us a little bit of how you get angry?

Betsy: As my sister, right?

Facilitator: Right.

Betsy: *(as Margaret, but falling out of role and speaking in third person as a narrative)* She can throw things and she'll stomp out of the house or she'll move out of the house. She would get a truck, back-up to the house, and move everything out. And maybe I'll feel bad later on when I think about it.

Note: The emotional intensity was such that the facilitator decided it was better not to interrupt her to have her go back to using the first person. She corrects herself towards the end. In the last sentence she refers to herself again, in the first person, as Margaret.

Facilitator: Maybe.

Betsy: *(as Margaret)* Maybe.

Facilitator: What kind of things do you throw?

Betsy: *(as Margaret)* Furniture, whatever.

Facilitator: And no consequences.

Betsy: *(as Margaret)* Ever.

Facilitator: You know what your sister was telling me. She was telling me that she had a lot of consequences.

Betsy: *(as Margaret)* I don't see it that way.

Facilitator: You don't? How do you feel?

Betsy: *(as Margaret)* I get yelled at a lot.

Facilitator: Uh-huh. Sounds like your sister said she got hit. Did you?

Betsy: *(as Margaret)* She did.

Facilitator: Did you?

Betsy: *(as Margaret)* No. No.

Facilitator: Maybe that's what she meant.

Betsy: *(as Margaret)* I wouldn't get it.

Facilitator: What would you do?

Betsy: *(as Margaret)* Probably walk out.

Facilitator: Uh-huh. I'm just going to ask you to stay in this role for a second. Are you okay with that?

Betsy: Uh-huh.

Facilitator: Can I ask you to choose somebody to be your sister?

Betsy: Valerie.

Facilitator: *(to Valerie)* Would that be okay? Why don't we reverse roles here, and, Valerie, why don't you come here and sit in the actual seat. *(now talking to Betsy)* And I would like you to keep a conversation going with me as we do this. Valerie is going to lose it. *(Everybody laughs.)*

(to Betsy) You don't have to pay attention to it, you're protected. We have a shield here. So you will hear it, but you really won't have to deal with it. It is really more like watching a movie of your sister. She really can't hurt you. And I would like you to talk to me while that is going on. *(now talking to Valerie)* So could you begin ... and lose it! *(Everyone laughs.)*

Facilitator: *(to Betsy)* What is something that your sister would lose it on?

Betsy: Well, how she does everything for my parents.

Facilitator: Does she go quick with that stuff, or does she build up to it?

Betsy: She's real quick.

Facilitator: *(to Valerie)* So about a ten-second fuse on this. And on a one-to-ten scale, bring it up to a three and a half, not too bad.

Valerie: I can do that.

Note: This is an inoculation drama. The idea is to take a somewhat tolerable level of annoyance and build up some psychological antibodies. In this vignette, the facilitator is asking Valerie to play the role of Betsy's sister, Margaret, at a somewhat restricted level. Margaret is capable of being quite intense, but in this drama Margaret is kept to a "three and a half" on the one-to-ten scale. In this way, Betsy is given the chance to develop skills to tolerate her sister's barrage of complaints and verbal attacks. The scene is set so that the role of Margaret presents a backdrop of constant complaints. While this is happening in the background, Betsy is asked to talk to the facilitator about what she is feeling and experiencing, with her sister's voice in the background. This allows Betsy to become more self-aware and more conscious of her own internal process. By talking to the facilitator during the sister's on-going monologue, she gains composure and a sense of relief. She has been inoculated to her projection of her sister's critical complaints. To clarify what is happening:

Valerie, in the role of Margaret, is seated facing Betsy. The facilitator is standing next to Betsy, who is having an ongoing dialogue with the facilitator. In the transcript that follows, Margaret's monologue is set in *italic* type. The dialogue between Betsy and the facilitator is in regular type and is inserted throughout the sister's monologue as it happened in the vignette.

Facilitator: *(to Valerie)* Begin.

Valerie: (as Margaret) *I've really had it with you not doing anything for Mom and Dad. I can't stand it.*

Facilitator: Tell me what is happening. Tell what you are feeling.

Betsy: I am trying not to listen, but I can't help but hear.

Valerie: (as Margaret) *I feel like I am the only one doing anything. You never do anything. I can't stand it. I am the only one always. I have to do everything. Ugh. I have to drive them all over.*

Facilitator: Focus on your own feelings.

Betsy: Anxiety.

Facilitator: Can you handle this anxiety at the moment?

Betsy: Uh-huh.

Valerie: (as Margaret) *I drive them everywhere, buy them clothes, and you never have to do anything! You're way over there, and I am way over here. I am sick of this. I get really sick of this.*

Betsy: I just don't want to hear it. I want her to leave.

Facilitator: So you won't have to hear it anymore?

Betsy: Uh-huh.

Valerie: (as Margaret) *Why don't you do anything? You're not really involved with this. I am the only one that appreciates this. You know I am not the only daughter involved here. I can't believe this. You don't have to do anything. I have to buy underwear and clothes. Why don't you do something for them? Why don't you do something for them? What am I, the only daughter? I'm not the only daughter, you need to take responsibility here. Really, I have had enough. I am so sick of this. I really can't stand this anymore. It's not only up to me. You don't do anything. You don't do anything. I do it all. Why don't you do anything?*

Facilitator: What I'm going to do is ask you to keep going at this level until it becomes almost mundane. You have to tell me if you are getting close to it. Just focus on yourself while this is going on.

Betsy: I can hear it.

Facilitator: Uh-huh.

Betsy: I don't want to hear it. I could take a little. But all I want to do is hang up the phone or leave. It's total complaints.

Valerie: (as Margaret) *I've really had it with you not doing anything for Mom and Dad. I can't stand it. I*

*feel like I am the only one doing anything. You
never do anything. I can't stand it. I am the only
one always. I have to do it all and you never help
at all. You don't help.*

Facilitator: And you are usually the target of them.

Betsy: She doesn't raise her voice when she tells me
about this stuff, but if I cross her that's where she
can be really nasty.

Facilitator: And that's what you are concerned about the most.

Betsy: It really gets nasty. And my mother doesn't know
what to do either. No one knows what to do. She
keeps saying that I do nothing.

Valerie: (as Margaret) *I have to do everything. I have to
drive them everywhere, buy them underwear, buy
them clothes, and you never have to do anything!
You're way over there, and I am way over here
doing it all. I am sick of this. I get really sick of
this. I am really tired of this. I can't believe this. I
take them everywhere. You don't have to do anything.*

Facilitator: And that is really in contrast to what reality is.
You do everything.

Betsy: Yeah. The way I figure it. They used to live by
me. My father fell, and then Mom had cancer,
and I had to do it all. There was no help. HEY,
THAT'S RIGHT! I did do everything. She was
nowhere around. WHAT IS SHE TALKING
ABOUT?! *(Everyone starts to laugh.)*

Valerie: (as Margaret) *I have to buy underwear and clothes
and take them everywhere. Why don't you do
something for them? Why don't you do something*

for them and be a real daughter? What am I, the only daughter? I'm not the only daughter. You need to take responsibility here.

Facilitator: You look like you are feeling a little better!

Betsy: Yeah. I can handle this.

Facilitator: Now you are much more in control. You look like you have a little more focus.

Betsy: Yeah.

Valerie: (as Margaret) *Really, I have had enough. I am so sick of this. I really can't stand this anymore. It's not only up to me. You don't do anything. You don't do anything. I do it all.*

Facilitator: Now the thing that I want to do is give you some power. To give you the opportunity to tell her or show her what you feel or what you want to say. Now whatever you do is going to be successful. So what is it you want to do?

Betsy: Tell her that I have had enough.

Valerie: (as Margaret) *Why don't you do anything? You're not really involved with this. I am the only one that appreciates this. You know I am not the only daughter involved here.*

Facilitator: Okay. So whenever you feel ready, you can tell her. In this drama, now she will listen to you. So whenever you feel ready.

Betsy: *(to Margaret)* I've had enough.

Facilitator: Keep talking. Just tell her why you had enough. As long as you talk right now, she won't talk. *(Margaret's role is silenced at this point.)*

Betsy: I've heard it all before. And it is your choice. If you choose to do all the things you do that's okay, but I can't.

Facilitator: Good. What is the last thing you would want to say to your sister for right now?

Betsy: The last thing I want to say to her? Probably the last thing to say is that I love Mom and Dad and I know you do, too. So what does it matter who does what, just as long as there is somebody there to do it?

Facilitator: Thanks. Okay. We'll come back to the group. You did great. Thanks.

Betsy: Thank you.

Note: The group now reenters a sharing phase. There has been a spin-off drama, which emerged from the original. In this situation, there may be sharing that comes from both the original drama and the spin-off. It is possible to have multiple spin-offs from an original piece of work. However, due to the late hour, the facilitator will not have time to engage in additional spin-offs. An analysis of the group follows the sharing.

Facilitator: What kind of thoughts and feelings are people having?

Melanie: I feel like applauding, it worked so beautifully.

Facilitator: Yes. It was really something, Betsy, to watch your body change. You could see a shift. And I knew you were able to feel a shift.

Betsy: Yes, inside.

Don: It seemed like you went from feeling, like, this total victim to really becoming yourself. It was great to see you stand up to her. There are so many people in my life that never shut up!

Melanie: Let me tell you my last phone call with my mom. "Hi, Mom." I never got past that, then the whole rest of the time she starts talking about herself. "My teeth hurt. I have to get my eyes examined. I have to go to the doctor's." And on and on and on. I never told her my whole life growing up. She never received it. She always told me about herself. She never knew what was going on in my life. She had one child. She missed out the whole time.

Facilitator: Who else can share something?

Catherine: You were standing behind the chair wringing your hands, then you were so calm once you started speaking up.

Ted: For me there were a couple of things. I can certainly identify with what you went through with your sister. I would try to rescue my mother and get annihilated. There were a lot of things going through me as you did this. My mother asks me how I am doing and goes right into her own thing. It is hard for me to shut off my own thing while she is talking about herself. She shuts off when we start talking about anything real. I learned from this that I need to tell her that. I need to tell her what it's like for me when she does that. I am getting better at a lot of things, but there is more that I need to do.

Don: Another thing my mother is famous for is telling my brother, "Tell Don that I was meaning to call him but that I just got busy" or whatever. I used to just plain shut down. It is really very different now with my mother because I learned that it has nothing to do with me. When I get off the phone with her, I don't get all turned up inside. I used to, but not anymore. It was a marvelous thing to watch you. There is a fine line between allowing yourself to feel the feelings and having those feelings cross the line into hurting someone.

Betsy: Whenever I would hear anyone raising his or her voice, I would get this feeling. That's why I would have such a hard time speaking up—raising my voice. This is a great place to practice for the real world. OUT THERE!

Facilitator: Rehearsal for life.

Betsy: It really is empowering to do it in here with the group.

Facilitator: It is an okay place to experiment, to try things out. If it doesn't work, you have the option of retooling it and doing it differently.

Valerie: Much of my childhood had horrible fights in it. Where the police came and things like that. I felt that if I got angry, I was becoming like my mother. But then I learned that I could think and feel and then respond. It was only in my head that I was becoming like her. My children never saw that. They didn't think ... I am really grateful now that my children will speak up to me and tell me how my behavior affects them. I am really glad that you did join this group.

Betsy: I really don't tell anybody about my life. Nobody ever knew.

Facilitator: So speaking up here was very different for you.

Betsy: Very. But I feel a lot better. It really does.

Facilitator: Good. Let's take a five-minute break and then come back for processing.

[After the break, the group returns for analysis of the session.]

Facilitator: What kind of thoughts and questions do you have?

Melanie: I noticed that when Don started his drama, he started coughing. He coughed during the entire drama, and then it stopped when he sat down.

Facilitator: Probably not an easy thing to talk about.

Don: That's very true.

Valerie: I have a question. When Don was doing his work, when you asked him to play the role of the double of his brother, he didn't really play the double. He didn't really say the words from the double. And I was curious if you were going to ask him to be the double and speak it in first person.

Facilitator: I think he could have. It wouldn't have been inappropriate to do so. But my thought was, and this is *very* subjective, that Don being his brother—he was kind of in and out of it. He was saying it both as his brother and as himself. He would say, "I feel" then "He feels." It is a little like someone who is bilingual. They go back and forth. I think you are absolutely right. He wasn't in the double—but at times he was. It didn't seem worth it to slow the process. I also think that was more of a warm-up for the greater drama to follow, so it didn't seem worth it to slow the process up.

Valerie: That's what I was thinking, too.

Catherine: When Betsy was in her place behind her chair, you said to try some different responses.

Facilitator: Yes.

Catherine: And you said "Let's try anger," and you didn't get any other response. Is that when you had to go to something else?

Facilitator: Yes, plan B. *(Everyone laughs.)*

Catherine: That was quick thinking!

Facilitator: I'll tell you what I was thinking. Since Don had just done his drama, and Betsy's was a spin-off from it, it seemed reasonable to expect the same basic format, a catharsis in the role of the double—which is what happened over there—would be reasonable to expect over here.

Betsy: Except I don't think when I am doing a drama.

Facilitator: I found this out. *(Everyone laughs.)* It just seemed to me that the groundwork done in the first drama would be reflected in the second drama. It's like looking at a branch and noticing it has the same bark, the same wood, the same shape, the same components. In my mind, I was thinking about constructing a similar dynamic. Using an auxiliary with an empty chair, fairly similar dynamics, with your ability to express more of the emotion coming from the double. However, it was clear, when some people are blocked and unable to touch an emotion, it may be because of something in the moment, in the drama itself, or he or she might be in a situation in the enactment where there may be some cause for hesitancy.

(turning to Betsy) But this didn't seem to be the case with you. Neither of those things seemed like they were going on for you. It seemed like this was not available to you. That this option was

not available to you. It had nothing to do with the moment, or with the drama; it had to do with a core dynamic.

So I went to plan B. If you get stuck in one place, you change the time, the place, or the role. It seemed like the easiest thing to do was to change the role. Put you in your sister's role. There wasn't enough time left for us in the session to change the timing of your drama, to make you older or younger, and the place didn't seem very important in the scene. So just changing the roles was the next best thing to do—perhaps to try and have you experience the anger there. In other words, to let you act-out by playing your sister's role. The hope was that this would liberate you.

Also a technical thing: You mentioned stuff about your father, when you said that his rage was inhibiting. What I got from that was that if I put Betsy in her sister's role *(now addressing the group)* it's not unlike her being in her father's role. Both Margaret and her father were abusive toward her. Now, what happens is that once someone has been abusive to you, and you don't have control over defending yourself against them, except with some internal mental process, you can't defend yourself physically. What happens in that dynamic is that you do the best to defend yourself, but you also take in the abuser. You defend, but you also incorporate this abuser as an introject. In other words, the fear becomes "If I get angry like them, I will become like them." This is the despised self—"the worst thing that could happen to me."

(talking to Betsy) It was a lot stronger for you with your father than with your sister. So I was thinking about these things. The antidote for that

is to play the role of the abuser in a safe, psychodramatic environment. If you get to play the role sufficiently, eventually you will recognize that the stuff that is inside of you isn't your stuff. That it is their stuff that was imposed on you. In playing the role of the abuser, under the right conditions, you are, in essence, separating the yolk from the egg. You are saying, I don't have to fear this element inside of me so much because I know it was an external role. This was my father, this is my sister. I don't have to be overaffected by it. It is their stuff. I don't have to be infected by it. I don't have to own it. I just have to be aware that I was victimized by it, but that I have a choice as to whether or not I get in touch with it, whether or not I act it out. And I have my own feelings package. "I am not my father" or "I am not my sister."

So the tentative theory in my mind was, that since it didn't work over there, we should go over into the sister's role, and any gain over in that role should be helpful. If the protagonist has the facility to go into and out of the role, you get in touch with the fact that it isn't so scary, and you develop some facility for playing it and realizing it is an outside entity. You become aware that the despised self is a role inside of you that was acquired from an experience with another person, usually a member of your family of origin, and that it is not something that you have to remain victimized by. However, if that kind of role reversal is impossible, it may be because you still are being overwhelmed by that person, the abusive person, the outside force.

I believe that was happening in your case *(now speaking to Betsy)*. I switched gears at that point to go to what loosely would be called "inoculation therapy." I put you back in your role, assigned your sister's role to an auxiliary, and let that role happen at a level of intensity that you could build up antibodies against. Just like when you get a vaccination. They actually give you the disease in a small enough dose that you build up antibodies. This is the psychological equivalent to that. We didn't start off with a ten. We started off at a level you could tolerate. We started your sister off at a level that was intense enough to let you know it was genuine—something to be reckoned with—but not so intense that it overwhelmed you; it kept you safe. I have lost track of real time, but it was probably not more than three minutes.

Betsy: More like three hours in my time. *(Everyone laughs.)*

Facilitator: Right. There was a dramatic shift in how you were able to tolerate that. Now you are not going to be so influenced by her. It is another way to go to get the protection and insulation. But it isn't the way I was thinking about it. I thought it would have been a catharsis in a reversed role to give you the release. This is plan B—just the other side of that.

Don: I was thinking about, in the drama you did with me, how different the double was from the actual. I had to be removed from it. If you had tried to make me do it that one way, I don't think it would have worked.

Facilitator: Doing a drama is like choreographing a dance. Cha-cha-cha.

Ted: It is amazing how this works. I really did see a change with both people. I am doing more in my groups because of my participation here. I am happy about having this group and my groups come together. I am going to take it slow. I like how you reinforced to just go with it, to experiment with using action in my groups, but to go slow. It seems to be working.

The group comes to a close and plans are made for the next training session.

Chapter 7

ACTION METHODS WITH LARGE GROUPS

Working with large groups provides a different challenge from working with a small group. The primary difference is that in a small group, the dynamics are more readily observable. The communication between the members and the facilitator(s) is more direct, and the opportunity for anonymity is greatly reduced. You are noticed more when you are a member in a small group. The large group, in contrast, is more diverse in its membership and consequently more of a challenge to monitor and direct.

LARGE GROUPS

Number of Members

While there is no hard and fast rule about what constitutes "large" and "small" groups, I consider up to 20 people a small group and more than 20 people a large group. It seems that as a group approaches the very limits of a human family, they become more of a crowd. On a personal note, my maternal grandmother was the 20th child in a family of 21 children. I fully admit that my

131

selection of about 20 people as the upper limit of a manageable group might have more to do with my own generational experience than any universally agreed-upon number.

Characteristics

There are three principles to keep in mind when you are working with large groups:

1. Large groups need large group movement. Be sure the physical space you are using will enable the group to get up out of their chairs and move around. Spaces with stationary chairs are very difficult for people to negotiate.

2. Large groups are noisy. A hundred people moving around make a good deal of noise just in the movement of their bodies. Once you add talking, you have a noise problem if the facility you are in is not prepared for it. If a workshop is separated from you by a thin divider wall and the presenter next to you is giving a lecture, you run the risk of being disruptive when your group gets loud. When you make your original arrangements with the facility or conference organizers, be sure to inform them that your presentation will be active and at times noisy.

3. Large groups need more time to absorb information than small groups. Plan to cover less material in the same amount of time you would have with a small group, or schedule more time for the larger group.

Preparation as Facilitator

Prior to facilitating a large group, it is best to overprepare. In most cases, a large group will be both a training and experiential group. When this is the case, you would do well to prepare a detailed outline and description of the major topics you want to cover. This lets the group know right away that you have prepared for the experience. The display of competence also helps in members' readiness to participate.

Be sure to include your name, address, phone and fax numbers, and e-mail address, as appropriate, along with your credentials. You also may want to attach a 3 x 5 card to the handout. At the end of the presentation, you can ask participants to put their name and address on the card if they want to be included on the mailing list for future trainings. This kind of practice development should be adjunctive, however. Participants do not want to be inundated with advertisements of services, but you want them to have the information should they want to contact you. Your primary focus, of course, is to facilitate a good group.

It is a good idea to begin with a brief introductory statement concerning the expectations and intention of the group. You can ask the members what brings them to the group or what expectations they have about the day. In doing so, you begin to elicit feedback and interaction from them. Any good speaker will tell you that audience involvement is the key to a well-received presentation. Strictly speaking, members of a large group experience are not an "audience." They start in a passive, audience role, but move to a more active role. They participate in the event at some level. This participation is to be nurtured and supported, as it will determine the success of the group.

CHOOSING LARGE GROUP EXERCISES

The most difficult thing about working with a large group of people is keeping their attention. Action methods are the best way to get members involved in a large group. There are many to choose from.

Spectrogram Technique

A *spectrogram* is a simple and effective way to get people to interact with others. Choose two ends of a room as polarities, and then define the polarities. For example, you might begin by saying, "Stand down here if you are feeling really great today—if today is one of the ten best days of your life." Then go to the other end of the room and pick the opposite end of the polarity. "Stand down here if this is one of the ten worst days of your life." The rest of the people stand in the continuum between these two polarities, which becomes a spectrogram, where people stand and chat with one another. You can direct that they chat with their neighbor to make sure they are standing in the accurate spot. This allows them to make decisions about where they stand in relation to other people and whether they are too far in one direction or another. This seemingly informal matter of chatting helps people warm-up to each other and to the process of talking and interacting with strangers.

This use of a spectrogram creates homogeneous groupings of members. In choosing a spot based on how they are feeling, people of like minds tend to congregate together. Once you have people of like minds gathered, you can change the questions for the spectrogram. This means to change the polarities. By asking other questions, you encourage people to interact with different people and continue the stimulating interactions. If you wish, move the polarities toward the topic of your presentation. For example, if your presentation is on family dynamics, you can change the polarities to: "If you have you been in the mental health field forever, go down to this end of the room. If today is your first day in the field, stand down at the opposite end of the room." Then start asking questions about family origin: "If you are happy with your family of origin, stand … " These questions bring the focus of the group closer to the topic you wish to present.

It is important not to begin with difficult questions that involve deep psychological reflection or significant self-disclosure. Starting your first movement exercise with the directions: "Go to this end of the room if you feel you have not been emotionally or verbally abusive to your spouse for at least three months. Go to this end of the room if you have been emotionally or verbally abusive to your spouse within the past week," is likely to send your participants running never to return!

The spectrogram is a deceptively simple exercise that has many advantages. First, it gets people up and moving around. They get out of their seats and begin milling around and talking with one another. The event takes on the casual atmosphere of a cocktail party without the cocktails. Second, it can be used with extremely large groups. Third, it is a way for group members to begin the process of self-disclosure.

As mentioned in Chapter 3 on *therapeutic factors,* there are two kinds of self-disclosure. *Horizontal self-disclosure* involves the expression of relatively safe information. It is the "chit chat" that we engage in day-to-day life—information about the weather, current events, and so on. Simple questions are perfect for warming people up to the interactive process. As you ask a series of questions with increasingly probing polarities, the process spirals from horizontal to *vertical self-disclosure.* The spiral funnels the group from the perimeter to a deeper level of functioning, greater self-disclosure, and deeper interaction. You can tailor the questions to the group so that they become more challenging and thought provoking. For example, after some warm-up questions have gotten the group moving around, you may deepen the process by switching to a question concerning the family of origin. "Stand on this end of the spectrum if you felt good about your childhood and happy in your family of origin. Stand on the other end of the spectrum if you did not have good experiences in your family of origin. Talk to others to find where you should be along the continuum."

This type of question never should be asked first. Use your clinical sense of the group to determine what questions would allow people to continue to interact and take part in the process. The idea behind the warm-up and the spiral is to ease the participants into interaction with one another. Put yourself in the position of the group members. If you were asked immediately to start talking about the difficulties experienced in your childhood, you might feel overwhelmed, resistant, or inhibited. It would be too soon for you to handle a question of this depth.

Here are some guidelines for using the spectrogram that will help to ensure its success:

1. Determine the objective of the group. If the large group is meeting only once, the kind of questions asked will be

different from those in a long-term, outpatient group that has been meeting for two years. The questions would be different again for a psychiatric, inpatient population or for a four-hour training program for therapists. Determining the objective of the group will help you to decide what kinds of questions to use.

2. Know the length of the group. A one-hour presentation to parents on the do's and don'ts of disciplining a child will require a very different use of the spectrogram than will a six-hour all-day workshop for couples. In some groups, you may use the spectrogram simply to warm people up and get them comfortable talking with each other. In another group, you may use the technique to begin the process of self-disclosure for working on more difficult material.

3. Prepare your questions ahead of time and be prepared for them *not* to work. Decide what questions in what order would be helpful. Then imagine you ask the question but the people do not begin moving—they find it too difficult or they don't understand the question. Then generate an alternate question that is clearer or less intrusive. The idea is to find questions that help you move toward your objective. The process can get sandbagged along the way, so you need to develop resources that will loosen it up and allow people to continue interacting.

4. Be prepared to stop, switch to another technique, or abandon the technique altogether. I have had presentations prepared for large movement activities only to find out at the last minute that despite my request, the room I had been assigned had stationary chairs. In one group I had never been with before, I asked how people were feeling at the conference. Everyone walked down to the positive end of the spectrum, leaving just one man standing alone at the other end. When he saw the group and the group saw him, there was spontaneous laughter by all. However, within seconds the man's laughter turned to crying.

Of course, it was necessary to stop the exercise. We came back into the group circle, and, as the man spoke, we moved into a *multiple doubling* exercise in which the people in the group said how they thought he felt. Ultimately this was a very powerful and insightful session. But it did require that I abandon my original plan for using the spectrogram. If you are prepared to stop, switch, or abandon the technique, you will be able to be open and sensitive to the needs of the group.

To summarize, if you are using a spectrogram:

1. Choose two ends of the room to make your polarities. There should be adequate space for people to walk between the two ends and mill around.

2. Define both ends of the polarity.

3. Ask participants to talk to their neighbors to assess the appropriateness of where they have chosen to stand. This also leads to homogeneous groupings.

4. Ask different questions (polarities) that move toward your topic.

5. Begin with easy questions for warm-up; then move to deeper or more provocative questions.

Face of the Clock Technique

Another large group exercise uses a face of a clock on the floor. This technique was first used by Robert Siroka of the Psychodrama Institute in New York City. Ask participants to imagine that 12 o'clock is to the north, 6 o'clock is to the south, 3 o'clock is to the east, and 9 o'clock is to the west. If you want, you can tape numbers on the floor or wall to make the image concrete. Next, ask participants to stand by the time of day they feel most happy—the time they enjoy most. Ask them to discuss with those closest to them what allows them to make their choice. As with the spectrogram, this technique allows people to gather and share information in a relatively safe way while grouping themselves along the lines of similarity. You can then change the question. For example, you can tell them to stand near the time of day when they feel most relaxed. Once you have done one or two of these exercises with the clock, you can make the questions more specific to your topic. For example, if the topic is spirituality, you may eventually ask: "At what time of the day do you feel most spiritual or most connected to God?" and "What time of the day do you feel furthest away from God or least spiritual?"

The spectrogram and the face of the clock are two exercises that enable you to move large numbers of people in a relatively short period of time into homogeneous groups.

Self-Disclosure

Eventually, you will want to help the group become more intimate. The vehicle for intimacy is *self-disclosure*. As people reveal more about their preferences and their life stories, they engage in vertical self-disclosure. Once the group members begin to talk about their motivations, resistances, and reactions, this self-disclosure deepens the intimacy of the group as well as the connectiveness and cohesion. The trick for the facilitator is to help people vertically self-disclose to the point where they are able to profit from the group experience but not to a point where they feel inhibited. If members in a group disclose too much too soon, they will feel unsafe, particularly in a large group. The facilitator must manage the self-disclosure in a way that provides safety for the group.

You can accomplish this by choosing topics and questions that are not too threatening. For example: "If you are very satisfied with your professional life stand at this end, and stand at the other end if you're completely dissatisfied." This question allows people to talk a little about their lives with some degree of protectiveness. It would be very different if you said, "Stand over here if you are completely happy with your spouse, and stand over there if you are absolutely miserable with your spouse." This question elicits more intimate reactions from people.

It is good to begin a large group experience with statements about self-disclosure and confidentiality. The facilitator lets everybody know that they are entirely responsible for their level of participation. Although the facilitator can request that people keep the material that is raised confidential, there is no way to ensure this. Participants must know that the aspects of themselves they reveal are not guaranteed to be kept confidential. This kind of a statement gives members the responsibility for and control over their decisions about participation.

Grouping by Sociometry

Once group members have been warmed up by the large group techniques described above, the next step is to break the large group into smaller groups. How this is done will determine the success or failure of the experience. The worst possible way is to divide the group arbitrarily: "Everybody with red shirts over here" or having people count off—one, two, three, four, five, six—however many groups you want. These methods for dividing the group do not take into account the tele of the group members, and you run into the problem of divergent members trying to connect. This defeats the warm-up and readiness factors you worked so hard to develop with the homogenous groupings of the large group movements.

A more successful method for placing people into groups is having people choose others based on criteria of self-disclosure. The following explains an effective way:

1. After the large group exercises, tell the members to choose someone who looks like he or she would be easy to talk with, someone with whom they would be comfortable talking.

2. Once they've made their choices, they put their hand on that person's shoulder and, if that person then chooses somebody else, they must travel with that person to the next choice. Doing this creates small groups that are interconnected.

3. Then ask the members to share with the person they chose what allowed them to make the choice and to ask the person who was chosen to share back what that felt like. This makes further natural connections in the group. You can elaborate on the process with questions such as: "Who looks like he or she would be an easy person with whom to talk?" "Who would be a safe person to talk to about something personal in your life?" "Would you be willing to tell one thing about how you're feeling?" These are all questions designed to have people connect with others they feel safe with while at the same time investing in vertical self-disclosure.

4. After this exercise, you can ask that people form groups in which they feel comfortable. Having people choose who they want to be with maximizes the tele of the group and adds to the potential of your group's success.

Activating the Small Groups

When you put together small groups, you have created homogeneous groups that are likely to evoke feelings of universality, cohesion, belonging, acceptance, and altruism, based on their self-chosen similarities. Having been prepared this way, each of the smaller groups is now in a good position to work. Your job as the facilitator of the larger group is to create a project or task on which the smaller groups can work within a time limit. Again, the major principle is vertical self-disclosure. One task is for members to tell their small group how this group differs from their family of origin. This begins a process of self-disclosure that is targeted at recapitulation of the family of origin—more importantly, it is likely to target *corrective recapitulation*. When you ask people to compare their experiences in their family of origin to a group that has formed within moments, they take their experiences from an historical perspective and organize them into the moment.

If your groups are going to be meeting for a brief time span such as for a half hour, you give them a few minutes to go around with your first question. Then your second project for them is to work directly on the topic of the day. If the group is working on increasing their spiritual awareness, for example, the second task might be: "What has been your primary obstacle in feeling connected to God?" For a vocational training, your second task would focus on concrete issues relevant to work, for example, "Have you heard of or had experiences that caused you to question whether sexual harassment has taken place at your job?"

Closure of Small Group

The final task you give the group brings their experience together in some closure. This can be done symbolically in action. For example, in a spirituality group, people could hold hands in a circle and offer a silent prayer. In a vocational training group, people could shake hands and share their work numbers. After some type of formal ending to the small groups, members return to the large group, where processing, education, or training can now take place.

Move to Large Group Training

The training or educational phase now has the undivided attention of the group. Members now are ready to attend to the material you have to present because of the experience provided. The action heightens their participation and makes them ready to respond to your didactic material. If you try to present much didactic material first, before the group is warmed-up, they are less likely to retain the information than if you present it after they have had some experiential learning.

SKILL DEVELOPMENT FOR
LARGE GROUP EXERCISES

1. In a self-study group of 20 people, take turns choosing polarities to be used along the spectrogram. Do this at least six times to see the differences in alignment within the group. Follow the above directions and form small groups after the spectrogram exercise. Discuss the reactions and value of the spectrogram and generate other

polarities that you may wish to use when running a group. As part of your discussion, decide how you would modify the use of your polarities for a one-time use at a conference, for a classroom that meets several times, and for a professional meeting of colleagues who know one another but are meeting with you for training purposes.

2. In a self-study group of 20 people, take turns generating questions using the face of the clock technique. Following this, discuss the different type of questions you might use if you were running a stress management program, an in-service training on family therapy, and a seminar on personal growth. Share these ideas with others in your group.

Chapter 8

ADAPTING ACTION METHODS

Despite the evidence of its effectiveness and recommendations by researchers, group psychotherapy seldom has been used with people suffering from mental retardation, chronic psychiatric disabilities, and those with a dual diagnosis. In addition, when employed with such populations, group methods have suffered from being little more than socialization or teaching forums. Individuals suffering with a dual diagnosis of mental retardation and a psychiatric disability usually have been excluded from dynamic and interactive group processes.

WHY GROUPS WERE NOT USED

Historically, research indicated that people with the above noted disabilities could not profit from insight-oriented interactive therapy because they lacked the cognitive abilities thought necessary for therapeutic change. Although many clinicians have regarded people with mental retardation as unsuitable for any form of psychotherapy (Hurley, 1989; Hurley, Pfadt, Tomasulo, & Gardner, 1996), there are many case reports on the effectiveness of both individual (see Hurley, 1989, for a review) and group psychotherapy (see Pfadt, 1991, for a review). Psychotherapy for people with mental retardation is most effective when a directive style and structured sessions are used (Fletcher, 1984; Hingsburger, 1987; Hurley, 1989; Hurley & Hurley, 1986, 1988; Hurley et al., 1996; Matson, 1985; Schramski, 1984; Tomasulo, 1992). Active/interactive techniques stimulate sensory and affective modes of learning (Hurley et al., 1996; Tomasulo, 1994).

A series of erroneous assumptions on the part of practitioners may cause psychotherapy to be overlooked as a treatment modality for people with mental retardation. Consider the following major suppositions:

1. Since many developmentally disabled people are not verbal (or have difficulty verbalizing), they are thought to be unable to produce clues to regulating their behavior.

2. The secondary disabilities that often accompany mental retardation (short attention span, auditory and visual handicaps, seizures, etc.) are thought to provide insurmountable obstacles to interactive group therapy.

3. People with mental retardation are thought to lack the cognitive ability to profit from insight into the causes and consequences of their behavior.

4. Because the emotional disorders displayed by people with mental retardation are seen as a side effect of a biochemical brain dysfunction, many practitioners feel there is little that psychotherapy can offer.

5. The emotional and behavioral problems of people with mental retardation are understood as being the result of either mental illness *or* behavior disorders, so either psychopharmacological *or* behavioral treatments are sought. The use of psychotherapy to mitigate these problems rarely is considered.

Finding someone knowledgeable and competent to deliver group psychotherapy to such populations is difficult. Although more providers are beginning groups and developing group skills, group psychotherapy is still the least often recommended and practiced form of treatment for people with mental retardation. In addition to the reasons listed above, another reason group therapy seldom is used for people with mental retardation may be the scarcity of research showing which methods are effective. Although there may have been indications that group therapy is possible, the volume of such information was not sufficient to offset the assumptions of practitioners. The time has come for greater attention to be given to group process. Using group therapy for people with mental retardation makes good clinical and economic sense.

USING GROUPS

People with chronic psychiatric problems have had more exposure to group treatment than have people with mental retardation. However, with the advent of awareness of the dual diagnosis of mental retardation and mental health (MR/MH) problems, the need for improved group therapy procedures has been recognized. The effectiveness of action techniques with inpatients with chronic psychiatric problems has been well documented (Buchanan, 1984; (Buchanan & Dubbs-Siroka, 1980; Cox, Taplin, Berry, Roine, Meyer, Hewish, & Saunders, 1992; Spencer, Gillespie, & Ekisa, 1983; Starr & Weisz, 1989.) Consider the advantages of using a group format.

Advantages

1. The skills needed to run an effective group can be taught to individual counselors in a brief period of time (two to three months for a novice and considerably less for the more experienced).

2. In the same time it takes to run a teaching based skill training group, a more richly interactive group can take place through facilitation rather than teaching.

3. More people can be served in a group format than can be served in individual settings.

4. Treatment in a group is sometimes more effective than individual counseling.

5. The cost to an individual for group psychotherapy is cheaper than individual therapy.

6. Groups may target specific topics (anger management, sex offenses, bereavement, job readiness, etc.), so that members can gain support from people with similar problems.

7. Groups also can provide interpersonal support from peers struggling with different issues.

Techniques

A long-standing technique in training, education, and therapy is role-playing. Role-playing is used in nearly every phase of human development to teach and model behavior. Parents use role-play, and children use it extensively during free play throughout early development. Within the field of counseling, specific and elaborated use of role-playing has been developed through psychodrama (Blatner, 1996).

Psychodrama is an action-oriented method that endeavors to express a condition or offer a solution to a situation through the combined efforts of a group (Fox, 1987; Marineau, 1990). Self-help groups and the use of role-playing in education and training derive from the psychodramatic method (Blatner & Blatner, 1988).

The use of role-playing for training, education, simulation, dramatic presentation, skill development, and therapy is so pervasive and so woven into the fabric of our society that it is barely recognizable as a science, art form, and acquired skill. Its natural process is at once so familiar and so agreeable that people use it in their programs without the slightest hesitation. They think, "It's only role-playing—I know how to do that." Therefore, the quality of most role-playing activities is adequate but lacks depth and breadth. Few guidelines have been established for the development of role-playing skills for potential leaders.

Psychodrama is a particular technique of group psychotherapy, developed by Jacob Moreno, as is described in Chapter 2. Over the years, techniques from psychodrama (which deals with issues unique to an individual's life) and sociodrama (which deals with issues that reflect a collective concern) have been used with people with mental retardation. Psychodrama and sociodrama theories (Blatner & Blatner, 1988; Steinberg & Garcia, 1989) offer the most widely accepted format for facilitating role-playing within a group setting. However the primary use of role-playing has been for role training. More specifically, these techniques were used almost exclusively for social skills training, not for counseling. Teaching and training were the aim of social skills groups, not facilitating therapeutic interactions.

Teachers in social skills groups foster interaction between themselves and participants rather than between and among participants. Because the emphasis is on teaching a skill, the attention has to be focused on the teacher/trainer. In the Interactive-Behavioral Therapy (IBT) format, the emphasis is on interaction among participants for the purpose of creating a therapeutic environment. Instead of a teaching/training model, IBT uses a peer support/interaction model where behaviors having therapeutic value are reinforced as a way of strengthening group processes.

THE IBT MODEL

In recent years, the Interactive-Behavioral Therapy (IBT) model of group psychotherapy has gained wide acceptance for use with people suffering from mental retardation, chronic psychiatric problems, and dual diagnoses. It modified role-playing, psychodrama, and sociodrama techniques to accommodate the unique needs of this population (Razza & Tomasulo, 1996a, 1996b, 1996c; Tomasulo, 1990, 1992, 1994, 1997; Tomasulo, Keller, & Pfadt, 1995).

Attitude

In the classic book, *Zen and the Art of Motorcycle Maintenance*, Robert Pirsig (1974) noted that the Japanese instructions for assembling a particular object start with the following sentence (I am paraphrasing): To begin assembly, one must have the right attitude.

This is very much the case with the IBT (and perhaps group therapy in general). The facilitator must begin the group with the right attitude. Your intention is to help members interact with each other at every level possible. Try to clear yourself of other issues and distractions before beginning the group and dedicate yourself to the above intention. If you can maintain this intention, the obstacles will seem less drastic, the unexpected more easy to cope with, and the reciprocal joy found greater.

Length

The IBT model uses a brief time slot—45-minutes to one hour or even shorter. It uses this brief format for four reasons:

1. It reduces the possibility of exhausting the members' abilities to remain physically and emotionally present.

2. It keeps the facilitator(s) focused on the task.

3. It fits into the schedules of most hospitals, agencies, residences, vocational settings, and schools.

4. It provides a standard and acceptable time period for third party reimbursement.

IBT STAGES

The IBT model has four stages: (1) orientation, (2) warm-up and sharing, (3) enactment, and (4) affirmation. It combines theoretically sound techniques for activating therapeutic factors from the field of psychodrama (e.g., Tomasulo, 1994) with some modifications specific to people with a dual diagnosis, specifically, the orientation and affirmation stages.

Stage 1: Orientation

In a group for individuals with mental retardation, many secondary disabilities, as well as the primary cognitive deficits, inhibit interaction among members. Poor eye contact, difficulty with short-term recognition or memory, impaired hearing, delayed responding, confusion, echolalia, inattention, distractibility, speech impediments, and hyperactivity are just some of the obstacles to interaction among members. For this reason, the facilitator engages the members in "cognitive networking" during the initial, *orientation stage*. Having members repeat what was said to them, turn toward the person speaking, and acknowledge what was said, establishes basic interactions between and among the group's members. If the members fail to attend to each other, any other therapeutic, corrective, or instructional goals within the group will not be realized. The orientation stage also provides a familiar beginning signal so that members will realize the group has begun.

This process of physically orienting toward the person speaking, looking at him or her, and echoing back what was heard begin in the orientation stage but will continue throughout the life of the group. Without such rudimentary interaction, therapeutic factors are unlikely to emerge and be reinforced. Thus, the orientation stage is characterized by the facilitator(s) assisting members to interact with each other and participate in the group process. This is the goal of this first stage. If the members fail to attend to each other, any other therapeutic, corrective, or instructional goals will not be realized.

Stage 2: Warm-Up and Sharing

During this second stage, the group members take turns making self-disclosures, and the cognitive networking begun in the orientation stage is continued. The facilitator invites members to speak about themselves within the group. The content of their presentations is of less importance than the process. In other words, the facilitator's concern is with the dynamics of the group, not necessarily what is said by participants. The facilitator pays attention to the nature of interactions between and among various members. For example, the facilitator may ask the member who has just finished speaking to select the next member to go. In such a way, members are encouraged to pay attention to and interact with each other rather than just with the facilitator.

The facilitator then will ask the participants to share something from their week. Once each person has had a chance to go, the facilitator then will ask the members if any of them has a problem on which to work in the group. During this deeper level of sharing, the members experience a greater sense of emotional involvement within the group. The group becomes more cohesive, and the stage is set for action to take place. The second stage of the group ushers in more intimate interactions between and among members. This is referred to as the *warm-up and sharing stage* because the group members are warming up to the enactment, to being together, and to learning from each other.

For over a year, I worked with dozens of comedians at the New York City Improv. Prior to going on stage, the more seasoned comics would spontaneously walk, talk, and act silly. They were preparing for their performance by getting themselves into a state of readiness. You notice before an athletic event the athletes stretch, bounce, and slowly get themselves warmed up for participation. Even your computer gets itself ready for the tasks at hand. Preparation is necessary for maximum effectiveness. In many groups, too little time is given to readiness. Leaders begin with the agenda without preparing the members.

In the *warm-up and sharing stage*, the facilitator invites members to speak within the group. As mentioned before, the emphasis is on process. The facilitator's concern is with the dynamics of the group. Has everyone had a chance to speak? Who has chosen whom to speak after him or her? Who has accurately heard what was said? Each of these concerns far outweighs the content of the presentations. Indeed the content of your group will be lost without sufficient preparation of the participants.

Stage 3: Enactment

During the *enactment stage*, techniques such as role-playing and the double are used. The issues presented in the warm-up and sharing stage are formulated into characters with the help of the facilitator. Although only certain group members may take part in the enactment, the entire group's focus of attention is on the action taking place. The enactment stage is the central feature of the IBT model.

People with mental retardation suffer from cognitive limitations; they need concrete examples and descriptions to benefit from therapeutic encounters. Using various types of doubles during group provides for this need through a graphic demonstration of support. People will usually stand behind and slightly to one side of the protagonist. During the doubling it is not uncommon for the double to show his or her support by placing a hand on the protagonist's shoulder. These gestures make doubling a natural technique for use with mentally retarded people. Below are some modifications that aid in using the double with this population:

1. The double may say just a single word or even a single noise to express how the protagonist feels.

2. The protagonist usually does not repeat the phrase of the double (as is done in traditional groups). Rather, the protagonist simply agrees or disagrees with what was said.

3. Protagonists with secondary psychiatric conditions (e.g., paranoia or extreme anxiety) or traumatic histories (physical, sexual, or emotional) may be too uncomfortable to allow the double to stand behind them. In these situations, the double may stand to the side of the protagonist or sit in a "double chair" alongside and in full view of the protagonist.

4. Doubling for profound losses (e.g., death of a parent) are not encouraged, as the impact of the doubling on the members may prove overwhelming, thus creating a downward spiral.

Within the enactment stage, a number of techniques are used to stimulate interaction among group members. One of the most useful of these techniques is the double (Tomasulo, 1994). This versatile technique, which is highlighted in Chapter 2, can be a tremendous asset in groups for people with mental retardation, chronic psychiatric illness, and dual diagnoses. Other techniques that can be used during the enactment stage include the empty chair and role reversal. These have been discussed earlier in the book.

Stage 4: Affirmation

Finally, in the *affirmation stage,* the facilitator validates the participation of each member in the group. This is done with specific attention to the therapeutic factors (Bloch & Crouch, 1985; Yalom, 1995). Each member is verbally acknowledged for his or her interactive contributions to the group. When someone displays a trait that is interactive and reflects a therapeutic factor, it is reinforced during this stage. In the transcript of an IBT group, which follows in the next chapter, you will notice an affirmation of Cindy's altruism. She helps people in the group and she is reinforced for this at the end. The reinforcer identifies in concrete terms the interaction between one member and another via a therapeutic factor. This reinforces the member's new social skills. It also helps slow the affective intensity of the enactment stage.

The affirmation stage signals the end of the group and serves to slow down the emotional build-up that has taken place during the session. The primary concern of a facilitator is to attend to the emotional needs of the individuals being served in the group. If issues dealt with during the session have affected participants in such a way that they need more time to absorb the elements of the session, the facilitator may help participants by providing additional affirmations. Affirmations help members identify the components of their participation that are directly tied to therapeutic factors. Most often the affirmation stage allows members to return to their normal routine with a neutral or positive attitude. Thus, the emotional involvement in the group usually peaks during the enactment stage and plateaus during the affirmation stage.

VISUALIZING THE MODEL

Figure 8.1 is a depiction of the degree to which a typical group may expect to have emotional involvement from its participants. Note that in a 45- to 60-minute group there is likely to be greater involvement as the group moves toward the enactment stage. The readiness of group members to take part in the action portion of the group allows them to have greater concentration, presence, and emotional involvement. In this way the format and process of the interactive–behavioral model lends itself to creating an opportunity for a teachable moment.

The affirmation stage signals the end of the group and serves to slow down the emotional build-up that has taken place during the session. The facilitator's primary concern now is to attend to the emotional needs of the individuals being served in the group. If the issues dealt with during the session have affected participants in such a way that they need more time to absorb the elements, the facilitator may help by providing additional affirmations. An affirmation can help members identify those components of their participation which are directly tied to therapeutic factors and other interactive features pertaining to their emotional growth. Most often the affirmation stage signifies the need to close down the emotional aspects of participation and allow members to return to their normal routine in a neutral or positive attitude. Toward this end, the emotional involvement in the group usually peaks during the enactment stage and plateaus during the affirmation stage.

IBT is different than other models of group therapy in which action methods are used. In other models derived from psychodrama and sociodrama there are only three stages: a warm-up stage, an enactment stage, and a sharing stage. The IBT model evolved from needs encountered with this population. In traditional psychodrama and sociodrama there is what is known as the *Hollander Curve*. This has a bell-shaped format, with the initial warm-up as the first part of the curve, the enactment stage as the highest peak of intensity and emotional involvement, and finally the sharing stage. Members in this model get ready to move into action during

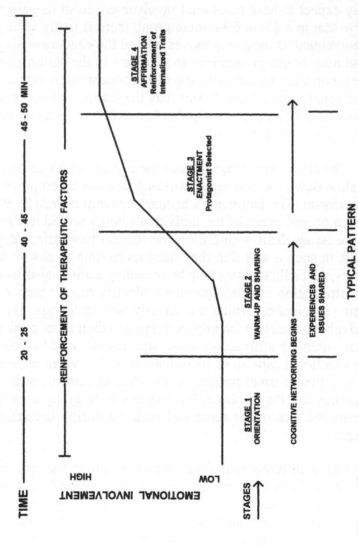

Figure 8.1. A typical pattern of the Interactive-Behavioral Therapy group process.

the warm-up stage, take part in an enactment in the second stage, and relate to the drama of the enactment stage by sharing in the final stage. The IBT model has an orientation stage first, to help members prepare for group process. The second stage collapses and modifies the traditional warm-up and sharing stages to allow members to express themselves, their needs, and their connection to the group earlier than might happen with a nondevelopmentally disabled population. Finally, there is the added affirmation stage, which helps the group end by affirming the members and halting the build-up of emotions.

Another model often used to describe action methods in psychotherapy is a spiral format with a funnel–shaped form. This model identifies the intensity of the session located in the center core of the funnel. The beginning of the session is on the perimeter, and the build-up of emotion continues throughout the session and moves to the center core. Typically, there is a catharsis or insight at this part of the group. Finally, after the core has been reached the facilitator guides the group back to the perimeter at the top of the spiral. The IBT model does not promote catharsis and insight per se, rather, it rests on the trust and safety in the group with strong peer support. As such, a spiral model does not accurately describe the IBT process.

In Figure 8.1 you will see that the IBT model follows an S-shaped curve, moving from lower to higher emotional involvement on the part of the members.

Emotional Involvement Through the Stages

The cognitive networking begun in the orientation stage continues throughout the four stages. This helps ensure that what is being worked on is being taken in by the participants. The orientation and warm-up and sharing stages are relatively tedious for facilitators. The task of weaving together the fabric of thoughts and words is often not very stimulating. However, this is the foundation on which nearly everything else in group rests. The time invested in these two stages is necessary for any return to be realized in the second half of the group.

Figure 8.1 depicts the emotional involvement of the participants in a typical group. You will note that there is likely to be greater involvement as the group moves toward the enactment stage. The readiness of the members allows them to have greater concentration, presence, and emotional involvement in the action portion of the group.

As facilitators, we must be mindful of the fact that the groups may stir emotions which may not usually be expressed in this population. Therefore, you want to be sure to provide an opportunity for each member to "decompress" from the group experience if need be. In these matters, it is best to err on the side of caution. If you suspect that someone has feelings left over from the group, connect him or her to an individual counselor, staff person, or teacher who can be helpful. Of course, the facilitator also may provide counseling.

Besides Figure 8.1, there are other ways to visualize the IBT model. It can be seen as a Hollander Curve, which is bell-shaped. The warm-up stage is at the bottom of the curve. The enactment stage, as the highest peak of intensity and emotional involvement, is at the top. The final, affirmation stage is indicated by the downward slope of the right side of the bell-shaped curve. Another way to visualize the model is as a spiral or funnel shape. The intensity of the session is located in the center core of the funnel. The session begins on the perimeter, then moves to the center. Finally, after the core of the session has been reached, you bring the group back to the perimeter. These models are helpful in understanding group dynamics.

Chapter 9

THE IBT MODEL IN USE

The following is a transcript of a complete session using the Interactive-Behavioral Therapy (IBT) model. The session, conducted in April of 1990, was the first in a series of five sessions run at the Young Adult Institute (YAI) in New York City for the purpose of making a videotape. Young Adults is a nonprofit agency serving more than 3,000 people every day of the year. The tape is used for training staff in the IBT model and includes a manual. The members of the group were unknown to the author prior to the taping.

None of the people participating as members had ever taken part in an IBT before, although they were somewhat familiar with role-playing. Each knew the other members' names and, in fact, all six members lived together in a group home. All were classified as dually diagnosed with both mild mental retardation and a psychiatric diagnosis. Members were offered a pizza dinner prior to the group each week. Their inclusion in the group was voluntary, and permission to record the group was obtained.

The group also had a cofacilitator, Catrina. Since the first group was designed for demonstration, the group was run more directly.

Catrina was more involved in later sessions. The videotapes and training manual are available from YAI. Their address and phone number appear in the Resources section, Appendix B, of this book.

The principles of the IBT model are demonstrated in this initial group. Each stage of the group is identified. You will notice that the facilitator takes a highly active, directive approach. Each interaction is encouraged and facilitated by the group leader. This level of involvement decreases as the group matures. Studies conducted on the IBT model have shown that, as there is less interaction between the facilitator and the group members over sessions, there is greater involvement between and among members.

This group characterizes typical initial group interaction. However, there is one thing that makes this group unique: All are residents from the same group home. This means they needed less orientation to each other. Usually the work done in IBT groups has a tremendous impact on the members. They get to work in a more direct way on issues they have developed during the course of the group meetings. Groups whose members do not live together have less opportunity to put their new awareness into effect with each other. They must transfer the skills they learn in the group to people they encounter in other settings.

In general, the process of psychotherapy reflects the evolution of awareness. Therapeutic changes in behavior are a by-product of awareness. The more aware a person becomes, the greater the likelihood he or she can initiate and maintain positive behavioral changes. Examples of this will be seen throughout the group. An effort is made to help people become aware of themselves as they interact with each other.

ORIENTATION STAGE

Facilitator: It's great that everyone is here. My name is Dan.

David: Dan?

Facilitator: Yeah, and I'm going to run the group with you for the next six weeks. You guys already know Catrina [the cofacilitator].

David: Noooooo! She's new to us. I've never met her before.

Note: The group moans at this remark by David because they realize that this is not true. Catrina is well known to them as a staff person they have worked with in the residence. Cognitive networking begins as soon as one person begins speaking.

Facilitator: So, what did you hear about this group?

David: Well, I heard this is a big chance to get into the movies and TV show.

Facilitator: Movies and TV show. Gretta, did you hear what David said?

Gretta: Yes.

Leah: I heard.

Gretta: To get into movies and TV.

Facilitator: Terrific.

Gretta: But I also heard that it was a counseling group.

Facilitator: A counseling group?

Gretta: That's what they told me.

Facilitator: Leah, did you hear what Gretta said?

Leah: Yeah.

Facilitator: What did she say?

Lenore:	Er, ahhrr, couns, er ...
Cynthia:	A counseling group.
Lenore:	A counseling group.
Facilitator:	Okay, good. All right. Maybe what would be good—you guys are listening so well—maybe you could just say your names so that we have all that on tape and we know who is who. You can just say your first names and that will help, will help me remember. Who wants to go first?
David:	Regis Philbin. *(laughter from the group)*
Facilitator:	Okay, but for this tape today we are going to call you ...
David:	Kathy Lee Gifford. *(laughter)*
Facilitator:	How 'bout we call you David?
David:	How 'bout Frank Gifford?
Facilitator:	That's a good one. Is David okay for this one?
David:	NoNoNoNoNoNOOOO! *(playfully)*
Facilitator:	We've got a bunch of names we can call you. Why don't you pick somebody to go next?

Note: The choice of who goes next allows for interaction between the members right at the beginning of the group.

David:	*(points to Hollis, sitting next to him)* Hollis.
Hollis:	Hollis.
Facilitator:	All right, Hollis. Hollis, why don't you pick who goes next?

Hollis: Catrina.

Catrina: My name is Catrina.

Facilitator: Okay, Catrina. And, Catrina, why don't you pick who goes next? *(she points to Cynthia)*

Cynthia: My name is Cynthia.

Facilitator: All right, Cynthia. Cynthia, why don't you pick who goes next? *(Cynthia points to Gretta.)*

Gretta: My name is Gretta.

Facilitator: All right, Gretta. You guys are doing great. Gretta, why don't you pick who goes next? *(Gretta points to Leah.)*

Leah: My name's Leah.

Facilitator: Leah. You look happy about that. You look happy about being here tonight. And, Leah, why don't you pick who goes next?

Leah: *(pointing to Lenore)* Lenore.

Facilitator: *(Lenore is slumped over to her right side in the chair. She seems resistant to taking part in the group.)* Can you say your first name for us? *(Lenore shakes head back and forth to indicate "no.")* Is it okay for us to call you Lenore? *(no response)* Is there an "A" at the end of that?

Lenore: Sometimes.

Facilitator: *(lightly laughing)* Sometimes?

Cynthia: She doesn't like her middle name.

Lenore: Don't you dare! *(group laughing)*

Facilitator: So we won't be talking about the middle name. So let's see what other people have heard about this. It's a chance to get into the movies—a chance to have counseling. What do other people think about the group? What do you think this is about? What do you think we will do here?

Hollis: Talk.

Facilitator: Talk. Good, Hollis!

Leah: I don't know. To meet people?

Facilitator: And to meet people. Did someone hear what Leah said?

David: To meet people, but we know everybody!

WARM-UP AND SHARING STAGE

Note: The members of the group have begun orienting toward one another through cognitive networking. Each phrase or group of phrases by a member is echoed back to them by others as a way of strengthening the communication loop. Once oriented, members tell a bit of their story. Usually members say what they have done during the week, as a way of easing into the material. There are usually two layers of information during this stage. The first is about the functional aspects of the week—what they did, what may have happened that was different for them, etc. The second asks the members if they have a problem to work on. You may ask this directly or it may evolve naturally as a form of self-disclosure. The process will be a shift from horizontal to vertical self-disclosure, from less threatening information to more emotionally sensitive material. Cognitive networking continues throughout all the stages.

Facilitator: Yeah, you guys know everybody, you live together. Well, one of the things I thought we could do as we begin the group is talk about what we did during the week. That way we can get used to hearing what people are working on during the week.

Gretta: Like what?

Facilitator: You tell me. What kind of things, Gretta.

Gretta: With what?

Facilitator: What did you do during the week?

Gretta: This week?

Facilitator: Yeah.

Gretta: It's only Tuesday!

Facilitator: Right! Well, how about last week?

Gretta: That's better. Like what? Inside the residence?

Facilitator: Yeah, inside the residence, at work.

Gretta: I went to work Tuesday. I didn't go Monday. I went to the doctor's. No, I didn't go to work Tuesday. I started work on Wednesday again. Then I came back and had a case conference.

Facilitator: Okay, let's hang on there a second. Who heard what Gretta just said?

Note: It is okay and even necessary to stop someone from talking to see if they were heard. Most members will respect this type of direction because for many of them being heard is a new experience that they want to have continue.

Leah: I heard.

Facilitator: What did she say?

Leah: She said Tuesday that she didn't come into work because she had a meeting.

Facilitator: All right, Leah, you are ...

Gretta: No, I didn't say that.

Leah: I'm sorry.

Facilitator: Can you tell Leah what you said?

Gretta: I said, Wednesday I went to work and came back and had a case conference.

Leah: I'm sorry.

Facilitator: Okay. All right. So you got it that time?

Leah: Yeah.

Facilitator: Great.

Note: Consider this brief exchange of information and clarification between Leah and Gretta. It allows the most basic communication principles of being heard and being able to correct misinformation to take place. Over time, members in the group come to anticipate that they may be asked to repeat or acknowledge what was heard. This increases their ability to listen more accurately.

Gretta: Then Wednesday night I did banking with my counselor. No, I worked on the banking with my counselor, but I didn't go in till Thursday.

Facilitator: Okay.

Gretta: Then Thursday I did do banking.

Facilitator: Let's just see who heard that. *(looking at David)* What did you hear?

David: She did banking.

Facilitator: All right!

David: Thursday. Right?

Facilitator: All right! Boy, you guys are listening great!

Gretta: Now I won't go back until Friday after work.

Facilitator: Uh-huh.

Gretta: Because my bank is open until 5:30.

Facilitator: Okay.

Gretta: And then I write it into a book. I have a behavior book.

Facilitator: Right.

Gretta: A hygiene book.

Facilitator: Let's see if Hollis heard that.

Cynthia: What did you hear Hollis?

Note: This is a significant feature in the group. We are only several minutes into the group and Cynthia has produced a spontaneous act of *altruism*—a significant therapeutic factor—by repeating my question to Hollis. She seems genuinely concerned with helping him respond to the question. There are several features about this that are important. First, it occurred spontaneously. It is a natural act that has emerged in the group without prompting or suggestion by the facilitators. Second, it provides the therapeutic factor of *modeling* for the group. The members are exposed to a cooperative act which is then reinforced. Third, it provides the facilitator with the opportunity to reinforce behaviors known to be particularly useful in facilitating interaction between and among members of a group.

Facilitator: Good. Good. Cynthia, you are helping him out. That's good!

Gretta: You know, I write in it at night. *(Now Gretta is helping Hollis.)*

Hollis: The book, huh.

Facilitator: All right, Hollis, all right. And it's Cynthia.

Cynthia: Yeah.

Facilitator: Cynthia, you really helped Hollis out there. That was good.

Gretta: And I want to say that on Saturday I went to my uncle's, and that's my weekend.

Facilitator: You had to go to your uncle's?

Gretta: Yeah, he's sick, but he's better now.

Facilitator: Okay. Let's see if Lenore heard that. Did you hear that Lenore?

Lenore: Humm.

Facilitator: Yeah, what did Gretta say? The last part.

Lenore: She said she go to her uncle's.

Facilitator: All right, Lenore. Boy, oh boy. Very good! That's terrific!

Note: I make a big deal out of Lenore's interaction because she was such a reluctant participant.

Leah: I heard it. *(Now, Leah wants to be part of the action.)*

Facilitator: All right, Leah, great! What did she ...

Leah: She said she went to her uncle's.

Facilitator: All right. A lot of folks are able to really hear you.

Gretta: They know what I do on the weekend. They live with me.

Facilitator: Uh-huh. That's great.

Gretta: Because when my counselor is not at work, Catrina takes my book.

Facilitator: Okay.

Hollis: Mine, too.

Facilitator: So, Gretta, why don't we do this. Why don't you pick the next person that will tell us about their week?

Gretta: Cynthia.

Facilitator: Okay.

Cynthia: All right. Um. I work at AHRC workshop.

Facilitator: Uh-huh.

Cynthia: And I do messenger work.

Facilitator: Great.

Cynthia: Um ... Monday and Wednesday I work at Project Mercury. That's like going to the various hospitals in Manhattan, Brooklyn, and Long Island. Sometimes on Wednesday I go to Long Island Jewish. What we do is ...

Facilitator: Hang on just a second. Let me see if Leah heard all that.

Lenore: I heard it. She went to New Jersey.

Cynthia: No, no, no, no.

Lenore: No, no, no, no, no.

Cynthia: Well, sometimes.

Lenore: Sometimes.

Cynthia: I go to Long Island Jewish on Wednesday. Parkway on Long Island Jewish.

Facilitator: Right, good.

Cynthia: I bring Medicaid papers to the hospital.

Facilitator: I see.

Cynthia: And sometimes they give me papers to bring back to the workshop.

Facilitator: Okay. Let's see if David is getting that.

David: She brings papers back to the workshop. Right?

Facilitator: Excellent. Good.

Cynthia: And Tuesday, Thursday and Fri, well, Tuesday I work with, um, like today I work with, Tommy G.

Facilitator: Let's see if Lenore heard that.

Lenore: She worked with Tommy G.

Facilitator: All right. That's good. That's good. Okay.

Cynthia: On Tuesday night the supervisor's daughter is out. So Tuesday I work with Tom. Thursday and Friday I work with Dora. My supervisor.

Facilitator: Let's see if Hollis heard who you work with on Thursday and Friday.

Cynthia: Who do I work on Thursday and Friday?

Hollis: Tom.

Cynthia: No!

Hollis: Who?

Cynthia: Dora!

Hollis: Dora!

Facilitator: All right! Good, and you quizzed him on it.

Note: Here we see a combination of therapeutic features. There is *self-disclosure* by Cynthia, followed by her act of *altruism* in helping Hollis. Hollis is also learning to listen better to what is being said. This is a form of *interpersonal learning*. The goal of an IBT group is to create a wealth of interactive opportunities during which therapeutic factors may emerge. Cynthia and Hollis demonstrate the spontaneous nature of the emergence of these factors. Acknowledgment by the facilitator reinforces behaviors that lead to positive interactions with people.

Gretta: He knows. He goes to the same workshop.

Cynthia: He knows. He goes to the same workshop.

Hollis: Shipping, shipping.

Cynthia: He does ...

Hollis: Shipping, shipping.

Cynthia: Receiving and reshipping.

Facilitator: Yeah. Why don't we have Hollis ... Do you want Hollis to go next? And he can tell us what he does.

Cynthia: All right.

Facilitator: Okay.

Hollis: I load trucks. I load trucks.

Facilitator: Right. In shipping and ...

Cynthia: Shipping and receiving!

Hollis: Shipping and receiving!

Cynthia: And boxes.

Hollis: And boxes.

Facilitator: Good.

Hollis: Um ... boxes. I load trucks. Ship out. I ship all the stuff out.

Facilitator: Super. Let's see if Leah got that. What do you think, Leah?

Leah: Hollis puts stuff into trucks.

Facilitator: Okay!

Leah: With boxes.

Facilitator: You guys are listening great. Very good. Hollis, why don't you pick the next person?

Hollis: David. Come on, David, wake up!

Cynthia: David! *(others in the background)*

David:	Yes.
Facilitator:	That was good, you guys helped him out. Tell us a little bit about what you do, David.
David:	I go to school every day, that's it!
Facilitator:	What do you do when you're at school?
David:	Cooking, arts and crafts, gym.
Facilitator:	Uh-huh.
Lenore:	You don't have to do gym.
Facilitator:	Good. Boy, Lenore, you heard all that.
Lenore:	We're related.
Facilitator:	Oh, you go to the same place? That's great. You really do listen to David. Did you guys work together for a long time?
David:	Nooooo.
Lenore:	Nooooo.
David:	A million years already.
Facilitator:	Already.
Gretta:	Two people who are willing to do things together.
Facilitator:	David, who are you going to pick to tell us a bit about what they do? *(David points to the facilitator.)*

Note: Within the field of psychotherapy there is some debate about how much therapists should self-disclose. In general, when asked for information about how your week went, etc., it is appropriate to offer a brief bit of information to satisfy the question then immediately bring the focus of the group back to the members. In doing this you remove the barrier between group members and facilitators, while putting the focus of the group where it belongs. There is no need to answer questions if you feel they are too personal. However, to not say something about yourself for fear that it would deflect from the focus of the group seems too rigid a response. If you return promptly to the group members, brief sharing by the facilitator is acceptable and can be helpful to the group process.

> **Facilitator:** Me! All right. Well, let's see. I'm a psychologist. *(sounds from the group)*

> **Facilitator:** Ugh, I ruined the mood. Yeah, that's what I do.

> **Gretta:** You're a psychologist.

> **Facilitator:** Yeah. I'm a psychologist.

> **Gretta:** Are you married?

> **Facilitator:** Yes. Yes. I'm a married psychologist. *(sounds from the group)*

> **Facilitator:** The worst kind, right?

> **Lenore:** Kids? *(Others echo this question.)*

> **Facilitator:** I have one child. *(Several people from group say "one child.")*

> **Facilitator:** I have one child; she's five and a half.

> **Hollis:** Wows.

> **David:** Does she ever need any babysitters?

> **Facilitator:** Why? Are you offering?

David: I love kids.

Facilitator: Yeah. All right.

David: Is she still in diapers, or is she out of them now?

Facilitator: No, five and a half; she's out of them.

Leah: I used to babysit.

Facilitator: Well. So you heard what David said.

Note: This is my opportunity to bring the focus back to the group. Remember the group is process driven—not content driven. The goal of the facilitator at this point is to bring the attention back to the interactions between the members. I am more interested in the fact that Leah heard what David said than I am in the content of what is being said.

Leah: Yep.

Facilitator: All right, Leah!

Leah: I used to babysit.

Facilitator: Terrific.

Leah: I babysit around my block where I used to live, in Brooklyn.

Facilitator: All right. We have a lot of experienced people here. I'm going to pick Lenore, because I really appreciate her being in the group, as I do with everybody else, but I know it was a little bit hard for you to come in, so tell us a little bit about what you do.

Lenore: Yeah, well, it's a little awkward to complain. I'm not going to complain.

Facilitator: I know you can't tell us everything because I am sure you do a lot, but could you tell us just a little bit.

Note: This technique recognizes that there is some resistance to participate on the part of a member. You agree that it is understandable that he or she wouldn't be able to say all that is going on, but that he or she might want to share a small bit of information. This usually helps move the group member from being totally resistant (because you have agreed with him or her) to thinking about what information he or she would be willing to share. The shift seems to be from an all-or-nothing decision, in which he or she is choosing "nothing," to a what-could-I-share decision, which often allows for some information to be offered.

Lenore: Humph.

Facilitator: How about one thing?

Lenore: Boring afternoon. Tuesday is the boringest afternoon of all. [It is Tuesday evening.]

Facilitator: Is that right?

Lenore: Yeah, compared to Monday, Tuesdays are boring.

Facilitator: Who heard what Lenore said? What did she say?

Gretta: Tuesdays are boringest afternoon after Monday. *(everybody chimes in)*

Lenore: Except for two things: One is that a lot of people yell every two hours.

Gretta: I don't really appreciate that.

Lenore: Yeah. Yeah.

Gretta: I don't like that.

Lenore: And, you really don't do as well.

Gretta: You don't get much money there.

Lenore: NO!

Note: At this point, almost everyone in the group has a reaction to the statement about not getting much money. They are talking about the sheltered workshop. There is seemingly universal agreement about the poor pay. Although negative in content, this is an example of the therapeutic factor of *universality*.

Facilitator: Lenore, as you're speaking I am noticing a lot of people are interested in what you say.

Gretta: That's because we used to go there.

Cynthia: We used to go there.

Gretta: And, um, like my favorite job that I used to do. I used to be a messenger. Okay? When I was in the Project full-time, and I was a very good messenger. Right?

Cynthia: Yes, she was.

Gretta: But I had a hip problem. So I had to go to another workshop. Well, I don't know what she *(Cynthia)* was going to say about me. I had to go to a new workshop and use some new work. I had to talk to a new supervisor last week.

Facilitator: Uh-huh.

Note: The interactions and conversation have become more spontaneous. The group members are drawn to participation. Lenore was not willing to speak only moments earlier. Now she is offering her opinion and has sparked an interesting conversation in the group.

Gretta: I couldn't take the new supervisor.

Facilitator: Well, you know what it sounds like we are getting into—talking about some of the things that bug us, and what ...

Cynthia: I want you to know that Gretta got a letter and five dollars at the annual Christmas party.

Facilitator: All right!

Cynthia: In December, 1990.

Gretta: Now you know that I've been out since then because of a hip problem.

Facilitator: Well, all right, Cynthia. That is very nice that you brought that up. [This is another act of altruism for Cynthia.] It sounds like ...

Cynthia: She got so many letters. And she got so much money for being on time. She was really a good messenger. She really was.

Facilitator: Let's see if Lenore got that.

Lenore: In December of 1990, she got five dollars and a letter.

Facilitator: Holy mackerel. Boy, you did great.

Leah: I got one, too.

Facilitator: We are getting to talk about problems, which I think we want to do. I just noticed that Leah didn't really get to tell us what she does. So if it's okay, we'll hear from her first. Then we'll come back and hear about the problems. So, Leah, can you tell us a little bit about what you do?

Leah: Yeah, I work in the workshop, and I used to work at Macy's.

Facilitator: Oh, yeah?

Leah: Yep. I used to work there part-time. Macy's. Part-time. I used to work at Macy's.

Facilitator: Let's see if David heard that.

David: She used to work at Macy's with the balloons, with the parade.

Leah: Noooo. Noooooo. Noooooo. Not with the parade. *(Everyone is laughing.)*

David: She used to blow up the balloon. *(David makes motions like he is blowing up a huge balloon.)*

Leah: *(laughing)* Nooooo. Don't listen to him. Don't listen to him. I was a packer. A lady packer.

Facilitator: Okay, a packer.

Leah: Yeah. I used to work in the fitting room.

Facilitator: All right.

Leah: I used to work in the fitting room.

Facilitator: Let's see if Hollis heard that. Hollis did you hear that?

Hollis: Yeah.

Facilitator: What did Leah used to do?

Cynthia: *(talking to Hollis)* Work at Macy's.

Hollis: Macy's.

Facilitator: Good, Cynthia, you are really helping out!

Cynthia: And, um, what kind of work did she do?

Facilitator: Good, Cynthia.

Cynthia: Packing, she did the packing.

Hollis: Packing.

Facilitator: Good, Cynthia, you really helped Hollis out.

Leah: I liked the fitting room.

Facilitator: And you liked the fitting room.

Leah: I liked that fitting room.

Facilitator: Okay, very good.

Leah: We got all the people.

Note: Leah is indicating that everyone in the group had a turn. This is perhaps a concrete level of *universality* or *acceptance*.

Facilitator: So you know how people started to talk about some of the things that bug you ... I am wondering if ...

Leah: I work in the workshop, also.

Facilitator: And you do the workshop.

Leah: I had two jobs before. Now I have one. *(Leah is eager to be a central part of the group.)*

Facilitator: Now one.

Leah: Now I'm looking for a job.

Facilitator: Okay.

Lenore: Another job.

Facilitator: Did you hear that, Gretta?

Gretta: Yes. She used to work at the workshop.

Facilitator: Oh, Gretta! Great!

Gretta: I was, er.

Facilitator: Gretta, it sounds like you have a problem you want to talk about.

Gretta: Two problems.

Note: This transition into the second layer of warm-up and sharing stage invites members to talk about more difficult problems that they may be having. Up to this point, the emotional level in the group is rather low. The conversations and exchanges have little emotional involvement. As the group moves into the second part of the warm-up and sharing stage, greater emotionality will be noticed. It is also important to note that although I, as facilitator, had indicated we were going to talk about problems, Leah's comments about her looking for another job and having worked in the workshop were accepted and folded into the process. It is at this point that facilitators are listening and looking for protagonists.

Facilitator: All right!

Gretta: The first one is, I'll tell you about the supervisor I had before.

Facilitator: Right.

Leah: Oh, yeah.

Gretta: Okay, this goes into the other problem. *(Leah is very excited to have Gretta talk about this topic.)* This is the problem. Last week I came back to the workshop on Wednesday ...

Facilitator: Right.

Gretta: And, like, she was getting on my case.

Facilitator: Uh-huh.

Gretta: Everything I was doing. I, she was throwing work back at you.

Facilitator: Oh.

Gretta: She really got me upset. Okay, this is how I'm going to do that—not next Tuesday, the following week. I will be in the hospital. Thursday, next week.

Facilitator: Uh-huh.

Gretta: And I will not make a Tuesday, for one week, and I don't want to be thrown out for that one day.

Facilitator: Okay. So you want to know if it's okay to miss a Tuesday for the group.

Gretta: This is a, er ... umh, this is a, er, I am having surgery.

Cynthia: She is. She's scared.

Gretta: Wait!

Facilitator: Good, Cynthia.

Gretta: On Thursday, after 15 years, I'm having surgery. I never had surgery in the residence before.

Facilitator: Okay.

Gretta: So, and Catrina knows about it because she was with me last week.

Facilitator: Okay. So you're a little bit frightened about going in for some surgery.

Gretta: And also because I don't want to. I like doing this thing. I like to be on tape! *(Everyone laughs.)* And I feel I have to go because I scheduled it already.

Note: Notice the depth of Gretta's sharing. As we enter the second part of the warm-up and sharing stage, there is greater emotional involvement. This allows for self-disclosure from others while moving the whole group toward the enactment stage. The facilitator now chooses a protagonist. (For suggestions on choosing a protagonist, review Chapter 2.)

ENACTMENT STAGE

Facilitator: Okay, so you're a little nervous. I have a way we could work on this.

Cynthia: How?

Facilitator: *(to Cynthia)* I know you want to help. And, Gretta, would you be willing [not "would you *like*"] to do this? To ... I'll show you how it works.

Gretta: Yeah, but, I was going to say, how is this going to help my problem?

Facilitator: Let's see how it works. Because I want to hear more about your problem.

Gretta: Why? What are you, a doctor? *(The group laughs.)*

Facilitator: I am a doctor, as a matter of fact. *(I motion for Gretta to bring her chair to the center.)*

David: Doctor Ben Casey. *(Everybody makes jokes about doctors from TV programs.)*

Facilitator: We're going to do a different kind of role-playing than you've probably done before. What I am going to do is ask people to think about what Gretta said about going into the hospital. Right. Now the spot right behind Gretta here is where you would stand and you would say how you think she feels about going into the hospital. As an example, right, I'm going to say, "I feel scared." *(turning to see Gretta's face)* Does that sound right?

Gretta: Yes.

Facilitator: And when I do that, when I stand here, you know what they call this spot?

Gretta: Role-playing.

Facilitator: Right, but they call this spot "the double." *(Everyone repeats the phrase "the double.")*

David: Yeah, that means you're going to stand in for her.

Facilitator: Yeah!

David: On the operating table!

Facilitator: Well, not on the operation! And since Cynthia knows you so well, Cynthia, why don't you stand behind her here. *(Gretta is seated in a chair in the middle of the group.)* Okay, I'll put your pocketbook down here. *(Cynthia is standing behind the chair in which Gretta is seated.)* Now Cynthia is in the "double" role. Say how you think Gretta feels. Say, "I feel . . ."

Cynthia: Er, Gretta, how do you feel?

Facilitator: Now you say how you *think* she feels.

Cynthia: Well, she's, I know she's scared about having surgery done.

Facilitator: Okay, so say now "I'm scared."

Gretta: Who, me?

Facilitator: Because you're trying to be her feelings. You just try and take it in, Gretta. You just wait there. *(toward Cynthia)* Say, "I'm scared."

Cynthia: I'm scared.

Facilitator: Does that sound right, Gretta?

Gretta: Yes, it does.

Facilitator: Okay, Cynthia, say some more, but say it as though you are Gretta.

Cynthia: I'm scared.

Facilitator: And ...

Cynthia: About having the surgery done.

Facilitator: Okay, does that sound right, Gretta?

Gretta: Yes.

Facilitator: All right! Let's give Cynthia a hand! Wasn't that great? *(The group applauds.)*

Facilitator: Cynthia, you did a good job. *(She returns to her seat.)* Now Cynthia did a good job of that. Lenore, how about you?

Note: This is the introduction of the multiple double.

Lenore: I can't get up. I have a bad back.

Note: Always offer an *invitation* to participate. Members must know that they are free to participate or not. Rather than see their refusal as resistance, it may be more fruitful to think of it as a need for another warm-up.

Facilitator: Okay, Dave, how about you?

Lenore: David!

David: *(He is getting up to go stand behind Gretta's chair, which is still in the middle of the group.)* Not David, Regis!

Facilitator: Regis, Regis! *(Now David is standing behind Gretta.)* Say, "I feel ... "

David: I feel.

Facilitator: How do you think she feels?

David: *(in a very high-pitched voice)* I feel beautiful!

Facilitator: Yes, she feels beautiful. And how do you think she feels about the operation?

David: *(loving the attention)* Happy? *(A number of group members say David's name with a note of admonishment for not doing it the right way.)*

David: Nervous. I feel nervous.

Cynthia: Scared.

Facilitator: Very good, and good, Cynthia, that you said that. Let's give David a hand. All right, excellent. *(members applaud)* So it was good that people know a little bit about how you feel. Who else wants to try? Leah, how about you?

Leah: You want me up there?

Facilitator: Yeah, how about we give it a try? *(David has returned to his seat, and Leah makes her way to the space behind Gretta's chair.)* That's very good. Okay. *(helping Leah into the spot)* And now, as you're here, say, "I feel ... "

Leah: *(looking to see Gretta's face)* How do you feel?

Facilitator: Now, how do you think she feels?

Leah: *(repeating her question to Gretta)* How do you feel?

Gretta: Nervous.

Facilitator: *(to Leah)* What are you going to say?

Cynthia: Scared.

Leah: Scared.

Facilitator: She said, "I feel nervous."

Leah: I feel nervous.

Facilitator: And scared.

Leah: And scared.

Gretta: And I feel scared!

Facilitator: Okay, good. All right, lets give Leah a hand, all right.

Note: All the group members applaud and they all seem quite happy with themselves. Gretta brings her chair back into the group. Now we begin affirmation of the protagonist. This happens at the end of the enactment stage and just before the affirmation stage. It is sometimes referred to as the "post-encounter affirmation."

Facilitator: Let's give Gretta a hand for doing that. Let's give her a hand for coming out. That was terrific. *(Everyone claps.)* What was good about what Gretta just did? What was good about what she just did? What did you like about it?

David: She brought all of her emotions out.

Note: This is from the same man who has been so oppositional in the group!

Facilitator: Yes, David. That's very good. Cynthia, what was good about what Gretta did? Because David said it was good she got her emotion out. What was good?

Cynthia: It's good she brought her feelings out.

Facilitator: Yes, Cynthia, good. Leah, how about you? What did you like about what Gretta did?

Leah: She walked out. *(pointing to the center of the group)*

Facilitator: Yes.

Gretta: I didn't walk out.

Facilitator: *(to Gretta)* Well, you walked out to the middle.

Gretta: Oh. Oh. Sorry.

Facilitator: *(to Leah)* Right.

Lenore: Yeah.

Facilitator: That was good. Okay. And you liked that part, that she took a little space for herself.

Leah: Yeah.

Facilitator: Very good. Lenore, what did you like about it?

Lenore: She was honest.

Facilitator: Yes. She was honest. Lenore, very good! And, Hollis, how about you? What did you like about what Gretta did?

Hollis: It's all right.

Facilitator: It's all right. She did good, huh?

AFFIRMATION STAGE

Facilitator: I think you did splendid today, Gretta. You know, because it takes a lot of courage to talk about that kind of feeling. And I think you did a terrific job with that. A really terrific job. How was it to have everybody say how you felt?

Gretta: All right. But, not next week, but on the twelfth I won't be here. When I do go, I'll be out only a week. I got to lay in bed. Even though I miss the whole week, right, I can come back?

Facilitator: You sure can. What do you say we give Gretta a hand for being so courageous? *(The group applauds.)*

Cynthia: But now I am going to ask you ...

Facilitator: Well, Cynthia. Cynthia, I need to interrupt you because it's time for us to kind of wrap it up, and that's an important question, and you can ask Gretta that maybe when the group is over, but what I need to say is I really like how today you were really helping everybody. I noticed how you were helping Gretta. That you were helping Hollis. That you helped a lot of people in the group today, and it was really clear, because I think that that is something that you work on. You work on helping people.

Cynthia: Yes.

Facilitator: So let's give Cynthia a hand. I think that that was terrific. *(The group applauds.)*

Note: Try to reinforce interactive behaviors of the participants. With Cynthia, I am acknowledging the therapeutic factor of *altruism*; with Gretta, it was *self-disclosure, installation of hope*, and *acceptance/cohesion*.

Facilitator: Hollis, today you were working on your memory. And I noticed today that, when you were trying to remember what people said, that as soon as people gave you a clue and helped you out a little bit, that you did a terrific job with that and that, you said it back to them and told them just how you were feeling. So let's give Hollis a hand. Right! For today. *(The group applauds.)*

Note: This reinforces *guidance* (from others) and *self-understanding* for Hollis.

Facilitator: And, David.

David: Regis, Regis!

Facilitator: Regis, Regis, Regis. You know what I liked? You know what I liked? Today you made us laugh, which was really great. That's a special gift, and you really made us laugh today. And yet, when it was time to be serious, you knew that Gretta was really being honest and sharing her feelings, and you were able to tell her that. And I think that you did a great job because you knew when it was time to be funny and knew when it was time to be serious. So let's give, who should we call you? David? Regis? *(The group applauds.)*

Note: This reinforces David's *interpersonal learning.*

Facilitator: And Leah you did a terrific job today.

Leah: Thank you.

Facilitator: Yes. You did a really terrific job, because what I noticed is that you were really working on participating in the group. Really being part of the group. I noticed today that you helped out right away. You got up and helped Gretta, and you were always trying to say that you heard what was going on. So you really did a good job in participating today. So let's give Leah a hand. All right? *(The group applauds.)*

Note: I could have said it more directly, but I was trying to reinforce Leah's *vicarious learning.* I should have been more direct that she was inspired to participate by watching others.

Facilitator: Lenore. You know what I liked? You didn't want to come into this room at all today. You took a long time to come in because the lights are too bright.

Lenore: Yeah, the lights are too bright.

Facilitator: Yet even with all that, you pushed yourself a little bit, and more than that, you listened to what people said, and you participated as much as you could today, and you did a great job with that. So let's give Lenore a hand. *(The group applauds.)*

Note: This reinforces Lenore's *acceptance.*

Facilitator: Now next week, we are going to meet at about the same time.

Lenore: I thought it was Wednesday.

Facilitator: No, it's going to be on Tuesday, about quarter to six. Now what we are going to do is, now that I know everybody's name and stuff, we'll do the same kind of thing and get to learn more about one another. Now you folks did a terrific job, and you should give yourself a hand for today. *(The group applauds and all get up to leave.)* See you guys next week, all right?

Chapter 10

QUICK START: BEGINNING AND MAINTAINING A GROUP

(A summary of material from previous chapters designed for those who want to get started *now.*)

The delivery of psychotherapy services for people with mental retardation, psychiatric disabilities, or both has made significant progress over the past dozen years. Availability, evaluation, and development of clinical skills for practitioners all are being investigated and discussed. Group psychotherapy is a central part of this evolution. It offers a unique vehicle for interpersonal learning. The opportunity for mutual peer support and feedback from interaction with group members is unrivaled by other forms of therapy. Proponents of group therapy argue that the depth, intensity, and capacity for change is greater than in individual therapy. While I am certainly of this opinion, more research is needed to substantiate the claim.

With the mandate to deliver psychological services to more people with less money, group psychotherapy may be more in demand. This trend may be accelerated for people with mental retardation. People with mental retardation are no strangers to groups. Indeed, it would be difficult to find treatment programs that do not include some form of group work. Although these groups are for social skills training, sex education, advocacy, etc., and are not necessarily of a psychotherapeutic nature, there seems to be a trend to include more groups with a therapeutic theme (anger management, relationship counseling, etc.). It is due to the proliferation of these types of groups that this chapter is offered. It offers a quick summary of how to begin and maintain a group.

There are many factors to consider in establishing a psychotherapy or peer support group. The suggestions below are not hard-and-fast rules, but merely guidelines for development. A group is a mini-culture. Every group has its own rules and rhythm and way of operating. Therefore, there cannot be absolute rules for all groups. Needs and conditions may be highly specific to a particular group. What works in one setting may not work in another. Group facilitators must be open to experimentation and allow themselves to make adjustments along the way in an effort to improve the functioning of each group. What follows are guidelines that many people have found helpful.

EXECUTIVE FUNCTIONS

There are a host of concerns which must be attended to before the first meeting. Group facilitators must make decisions about the group before it begins. The following list of issues should be addressed before your first meeting.

1. Establishing the role of the facilitator

2. Where the group meets

3. When the group meets

4. Who is in the group

5. Who is terminated

6. Establishing rules of the group

7. How many sessions will run

8. Who pays for group sessions

9. Adding new members to the group

10. Identifying the limits and requirements of confidentiality

Establishing the Role of the Facilitator

It is important to make your role as group facilitator clear and separate from any other roles you may serve in the lives of group members. Site selection can help in this process. For example, it is difficult for a manager of a residential agency to serve also as a facilitator for a group of residents. The residential manager often has to administer restrictions and limitations. The facilitator, on the other hand, has to create a safe and supportive atmosphere. While it may be argued that the goals are similar, if not identical, the manner and style of reaching them are very different. As such, the residential manager who becomes a facilitator may compromise both roles. He or she may have to carry out a contingency for a behavior management plan with a resident only a half an hour before having that same resident in a group. The shift in roles will be confusing and possibly impossible for the resident to adjust to adequately.

Preventing dual roles is a concern common to most therapeutic situations (e.g., teachers cannot simultaneously be their students' therapists), and this restriction should be extended to the running of groups in facilities where, due to the diversity and complexity of the job duties, dual roles may be overlooked or not acknowledged.

One solution to this dilemma is never to run a group in the place where you work. Establish a group at another work site within the agency or at another agency altogether. This may help prevent burnout for the facilitator, as it keeps the time, setting, membership, and role definition separate from the usual routine. It may provide the facilitator with clearly defined responsibilities and a sense of empowerment, two components known to reduce the potential of burnout. Being an "outside" facilitator has the additional advantage of enhancing the status and effectiveness of the group. Although status is most likely enhanced by the *Hawthorne Effect* (people feeling valued by the special arrangements made to help them), the group members tend to feel safer when the facilitators do not have a dual role, as issues of confidentiality within the group are less pronounced.

It may not, however, always be possible to separate the facilitator's roles. When this is the case, the following suggestions are offered:

1. Provide a clear explanation of the different roles served in the lives of group members. The group facilitator's job is to help members understand their feelings and solve problems. Explain how this may differ from other responsibilities during other times of the day.

2. Anticipate that it may be difficult for some members of the group to distinguish the different roles of the facilitator and that this may cause inhibition. If members can acknowledge this situation, ask if there is anything you can do that would help them. Some possibilities are to assure confidentiality and to clarify the goals of the group. The facilitator can explain that members may participate in the group on a trial basis, where members can test out how it feels to be in the group for two or three sessions.

3. If a member shows persistent signs of inhibition and discomfort, offer to arrange for participation in another group or offer individual counseling as an alternative.

Where the Group Meets

The meeting room should have privacy, adequate ventilation, and seating in a circle for three more people than you plan to have. There should be no chairs or tables in front of members when they sit in the circle. These will block work in the group, particularly if action techniques, such as role-playing, are employed. The chairs should be durable, firm, yet not overly comfortable. Too much comfort inhibits group work, too little distracts. The close proximity of a restroom and water cooler provides the group with physical comfort. Safety is another important consideration. Take care that security, including proper lighting of the room and building hallways, is provided during times the group is in session. The availability of a phone (for emergencies) and knowledge of the electrical panel (to reset circuit breakers) are useful. While these concerns may seem trivial, experience has shown that each can be a cause for concern.

When the Group Meets

The timing of groups varies greatly, but many programs find an hour to be sufficient, with a regular and definite starting time. Some programs prefer weekly meetings. Other programs run two brief groups twice a day. Some high-functioning day programs find a weekly format sufficient. Some day activity programs with polydiagnostic individuals functioning at low levels may find that briefer, more structured groups increase members' participation and awareness. There is no right or wrong length or frequency. Each situation is different, and the facilitator must decide what suits the needs and mission of the program.

Who Is in the Group

If facilitating a group is a relatively new experience for you, limit the group to a total of six members. This will keep your energy level from being depleted. Keep in mind that, as the facilitator, you have a host of executive and clinical functions to manage during the group. For example, the many tasks listed here have to be balanced with actually running the group and managing the group's dynamics!

If your first group experience is not positive, you will be less likely to continue in the role of group facilitator. If this is a beginning experience, choose group members you like, who are easy to work with, and who say they are willing to work with you in a group. Remember that sociometry is an important tool in healing. Facilitating people with whom you have a positive connection will allow you to assimilate new skills and develop confidence in supporting group process. After the first group, you will be able to extend your skills to groups with more complex and difficult needs.

Who Is Terminated

Termination of members may be based on a wide variety of criteria. It may be necessary to remove a person from the group who is significantly deviant from the norm. The term *deviance* does not here refer to pathology. The highest functioning member in a group of less capable people may be better served by moving to another group. No formula has been devised for removing people. Someone may be removed from a group because of persistent and unacceptable hygiene.

One group member complained that no one else in the group had a girlfriend. He asked to join a group with people who had the same issues as he did—a request that was granted. When a request to change groups is made, it is important to evaluate the reasons, both stated and unstated, for the request. One group member who was doing well suddenly insisted that he switch groups. When the reason was explored, it was found out that he owed someone in group a dollar and did not have the money. In this case, the facilitator encouraged the two of them to work it out in the group. They did: payment of $.25 a week for a month. Members who are too pathological for the group to tolerate may be removed and referred for individual therapy or, if the situation warrants it, for a psychological or psychiatric evaluation.

Establishing Rules of the Group

The rules of the group may be quite simple, such as: "No one can hit anyone else in group." Or they might be more elaborate: "People coming to group must be on time, be prepared with an issue to discuss, and keep the discussions in the group private." It is the responsibility of the facilitator to identify the rules of the group. However, not all rules will be immediately clear in the beginning. For example, the rule, "No singing before group starts," was established in a school where the singing became routine and was too loud.

In addition, it is important to be flexible with rules. Typically, facilitators make a point of saying that members have to stay in the group unless they have to go to the bathroom. This rule was amended during a group in which a member became so distraught that she felt compelled to leave. After following up to make sure the member was all right, the facilitator returned to the group. About five minutes later, the member returned. The facilitator immediately praised her for having the sense to know that she needed to take a moment for herself, and, in the same sentence, praised her for the fact she returned: "It was OK that you left because of what you were feeling. It was even better that you allowed yourself to come back." This established a new rule—with some flexibility to it. On subsequent occasions, people who left, returned. This helped prevent acting out on the part of members who would have had difficulty remaining.

How Many Sessions Will Run

Facilitators must experiment with time and frequency to determine effectiveness. In order to become familiar with the group and to develop facilitation skills, an initial run of six to twelve sessions is generally ideal. Once the group is ongoing, the facilitator can post a schedule so people know when the group is going to take place. Of course, provisions for canceling a meeting because of bad weather or illness of the facilitator are needed.

Who Pays for the Group Sessions

Private practitioners and professionals who work in a facility that needs outside funding must find ways to finance group work. There are five primary ways to fund a group.

1. *Private fees.* Some people may have the means to pay. As long as this policy does not interfere with other insur-

ances a member may have or with agency policy, private funding may be a possibility.

2. *Vocational rehabilitation voucher.* These vouchers are applicable when the purpose of the group is job readiness or job training.

3. *The State Division of Mental Retardation, or Mental Health, or Division of Developmental Disabilities.* Sometimes a state agency is willing to sponsor group counseling for the people it serves.

4. *Health insurance.* Medicare/Medicaid and other insurance billing is possible in many situations.

5. *Offer services for free.* When possible, group counseling skills should be offered to those who would not be able to have the service if they had to pay. One way to do this is to keep a number of time slots available for no fee services. When these slots are vacant, let the local agencies know and screen the most appropriate candidates for the groups.

Adding New Members to the Group

As new members are added, the volume of information and the interactive elements of the group (such as noticing therapeutic factors) increase exponentially. For example, the addition of one other male to a group of five women and one male changes the sociometry (the measure of the strength of interaction between and among people) in a way that is different from when one female joins a previously all male group. The addition of this member may change how individuals relate to one another and how they express themselves. For example, a woman joined a group of men who, for reasons only of circumstance, had not had a woman in the group for six months. It was immediately noticeable that cursing in the group stopped and two of the members began combing their hair before sessions—behavior that was completely absent from their preparations prior to her joining.

Identifying the Limits and Requirements of Confidentiality

Confidentiality is an important aspect of group work, however, it can be difficult to maintain in groups run in agencies and hospitals. The difficulties have to do with different mandates. For example, two professionals, each from a different discipline, running a group for an agency, had conflicting requirements for confidentiality from their professions, the agency, and the state they were working in. Check specific guidelines with each agency, state, and profession before beginning a group. This is particularly important if group members are from high risk populations such as sexual offenders.

In any group, it is important to establish guidelines for confidentiality between and among the members. Specific instructions about confidentiality should be given to members at the first meeting. For example, you might inform the group: "What we say to each other here is to be kept private. For this to be the kind of group where people can trust one another and feel safe with one another, we all must agree that we are not going to talk to other people outside the group about what we talk about inside the group." Members in the group should then be given examples. "Harriet, if Jane told us that someone bothered her at the bus stop and she got very scared, do you think it would be okay for you to tell that to someone outside this group?" This would then lead to a group discussion of the need for information to be kept private, which might take the major part of the first session. It should be noted that it is better to refer to the confidentiality of the group by using words like "private" or "personal" rather than "secret," as the keeping of "secrets" is more likely to be linked with sexual or otherwise inappropriate behavior than with a healthy respect for one's rights.

Once you are reasonably assured that the members understand the confidential nature of the group, you may then help them understand the proper way to take information out of the group. In returning to the above example, you might then say: "What if Harriet were angry about what happened to Jane and she wanted to talk about it with someone outside of the group? How would she do that?" At this point you would help the group to understand the basic principals of confidentiality. These are:

1. Do not use the name of the group member who said something that you want to talk about.

2. Talk about your own reaction to what was said, not the situation or the story of the member who said it.

3. Talk only about yourself, not about others in the group.

Next, it should be made clear that as facilitator you cannot guarantee that everyone in the group will keep things private. But you do guarantee that if you learn that someone is exposing what people say outside of group, you will ask them to leave.

Finally, you should let the members know the limits of your and your cofacilitator's confidentiality. As mentioned earlier, requirements may be different from profession to profession and agency to agency, but generally if you are told or suspect that a member in the group is going to hurt or abuse someone (or were hurt or abused by someone) you would need to tell someone else about it. This should be explained to the group members. Again, concrete examples and questions for discussion would be appropriate.

A gray area of confidentiality resides in communication between the facilitator(s) and other staff and family involved with the participant. Most often individuals are referred to a group based on needs assessed by others. The work done in group is often part of an Individual Habilitation Plan (IHP), an Individual Educational Plan (IEP), or some other developmentally organized plan or review. As such, the facilitator(s) will be asked to give feedback on and insight into the "progress" of the individual.

The term "progress" is noted in quotes because not all groups need to have clear behavioral goals with specific, measurable outcomes. It would be entirely appropriate, and perhaps necessary, for a group to exist solely as a support for its members' mutual caring of each other. That is to say, a member could come to the group, effectively use the group, and be an integrated member of the group for no other reason than he or she needed to be heard and understood. The "progress" of this person would not necessarily be measured in the form of behavioral checklists. Rather, he or she simply may be understood as a member in a group where the safety and acceptance he or she experiences may not be matched in other areas of his or her life.

When a request for information is made of the facilitator(s), it is incumbent upon them to inform the participant of the request and get permission. In this way, the integrity of the group's dynamics and respect for the individual are observed. If the information is of a particularly sensitive nature, a written release should be obtained.

ENHANCING GROUP LEADER SKILLS

Cofacilitation

Working with a cofacilitator provides opportunities to help one another develop skills. When getting ready to run a group, you feel excitement as well as anxiety about doing well. A cofacilitator with whom you share enjoyment and enthusiasm can help establish a positive learning environment for both facilitators and group members. Cofacilitators working well together in a cooperative fashion serve as role models for the group.

After sessions, cofacilitators can review videotapes, discuss process, and generate alternatives. This is extremely helpful in continuing the development of your group facilitation skills.

Evaluation

Most groups, such as those that exist in day programs, meet weekly. In some specialized settings, such as inpatient programs, groups may meet two to five times a week. Whatever the frequency of meetings, it is important to establish a point for reviewing the work of the group. For the first group you run, after the twelfth session, stop to identify problems in the group, notice strengths, and determine your direction. While cofacilitators should meet at least briefly after each group, an established evaluation point ensures time to reflect and evaluate the process and effectiveness of the group.

Videotape

You should videotape as many group sessions as possible when you are beginning to facilitate groups, but first you must secure signed and valid releases from all members or from their legal guardians. Videotapes provide a record of the group and give you an opportunity to assess the effectiveness of the group over time. Videotapes also let you track the emergence of therapeutic factors. For example, when a usually volatile member of the group hands a another member who is crying a box of tissues, showing a videotape of this spontaneous act of *altruism* highlights to the individual his or her own individual positive behavior. This is a particularly potent way to promote learning through modeling (i.e., self-modeling).

To elaborate on the above technique, you may use edited versions of videotapes to create a positive self-model for selected members of the group. For this procedure, scan the videotape for a desirable interaction that may occur infrequently with a group member. Edit the videotape to show an extended segment with the member displaying a trait you hope to have occur more often. Be sure to tape the affirmation of the trait in the original video and add this to the end of the segment.

> **Case of Victor.** It was determined that Victor needed help with direct eye contact while talking to someone. He very rarely looked at anyone in the group and often stared at the floor. On the rare occasions when he was looking up, he was praised immediately for his action. This was captured on video over several sessions, so we were able to put together about a two minute segment of Victor looking directly at the people who were talking

or with whom he was talking. Victor was shown this as part of a video feedback group and in individual sessions. In tracking his progress, we noted that he was able to look directly at people for longer periods of time after we had shown him the tape. Indeed, the tape became so desirable to Victor that we made others for him to reinforce other interactive behaviors.

In addition, facilitators can identify on videotapes missed opportunities for using different techniques. And, of course, videotapes can be used in training others in group process.

Processing the Group

Perhaps the biggest advantage of conducting a group with a cofacilitator is the opportunity to process and review the content of the sessions. This review includes watching the videos, talking about what could be done differently, and, most importantly, noting what was *good* about facilitator interactions during the group. Each facilitator serves as teacher and validator for the other. The following are important questions to ask during the processing of the group.

1. What were the highlights of the group over the time of the sessions?

2. What were the difficult points during the group? How might you have handled things differently during these difficult times?

3. Who profited most in the group and why?

4. Who was the most deviant (from the group norm) person in the group? Was his or her deviance such that he or she did not succeed as well in the group as you would have hoped?

5. What therapeutic factors emerged during the group process? Did some factors emerge more than others?

6. How did you and your cofacilitator operate during the group? Are there things you can do to enhance your cofacilitation?

7. Was the supervision you received adequate? What additional training, supervision, or reading material is needed to ensure your group's therapeutic functioning?

8. Was the space suitable? Was there sufficient privacy? Was the physical setting conducive to the development of therapeutic factors?

9. How has the group changed members' behavior outside of group?

10. What feedback was received from staff, parents, employers, etc. on the changes that have taken place with the members? What are others saying about the group?

Peer Support/Supervision Group

A peer support/supervision group with professional colleagues is essential. Most facilitators have found that starting a peer support/supervision group to discuss ongoing issues, problems, and successes with their groups is extremely helpful for long-term work. In general, a monthly meeting (at minimum) is in order. Such a forum allows each facilitator to share techniques and solutions with other facilitators. A variety of formats are instructive. Facilitators may review videotapes from each others' groups. One person can make a presentation on a particular therapeutic concept or technique. At other meetings, a guest speaker on a topic of interest may be invited.

Supervision

Receiving supervision from someone experienced in group process and how it relates to the population of your group is vital. More and more professionals are using groups for people with developmental disabilities and mental health needs. Professionals with expertise in a variety of areas are connected with various organizations. A list of organizations offering this type of training appears in Appendix B, Resources.

Training and Skill Development

To enhance your skills as a group therapist, attend trainings, read articles, and review training videos that pertain to your group. State organizations on developmental disabilities and national associations in counseling, psychodrama, psychology, human services, education, and behavior management have all offered workshops on the use of group counseling. A list of these organizations appears in Appendix B, Resources. Call or write to have them put you on a mailing list for their conferences. Training videos in group counseling are offered by a few professional organizations.

Stimulating Interaction

When there is no interaction among members of a therapy group or if they seem to be bored, most new facilitators feel pressure to do something to save the group from terminal boredom. Here are four different strategies to employ when the group is stuck:

1. You can get information about problems and issues that have come up for members during the week. If the group is made up of an inpatient population or residents of a facility, you can ask for this information directly from the program supervisor. You then can use this information to help activate a discussion of the incident or issue.

2. You can make a process comment to the group that acknowledges the fact that you recognize the silence (or boredom or inattention, etc.) and brings responsibility for it back to the group: "I notice that people are looking (bored, tired, angry, uninterested, etc.), and since this is your group, I was wondering what you might like to do about it?" This does two things: First, it lets group members know that the facilitator recognizes the problem. Second, it tells members that it is something for which they are responsible.

3. You also can become the voice of the group: "If I were going to say how this group feels, I would say, 'I'm tired; I don't want to be here today.'" This statement gives members in the group an opportunity to react. I like this method because it gives the members a match-to-sample with their feelings rather than a fill-in-the-blank task. Action methods such as a group double also may help stimulate a discussion. Even if you are wrong about your supposition regarding feelings in the group, members will correct it and a discussion will begin.

4. Perhaps the most obvious, yet most underused, intervention is to validate the noncrisis mode of the group. When people in the group are bored and the group is not engaged emotionally, you can acknowledge the lack of turmoil, the lack of conflict in their lives. Generally, this is a short phase, and members will be discussing their conflicts in short order.

The tasks to be managed when running a group cover a broad spectrum. At one end are the functional elements: Where are the chairs? The extra light bulbs? The circuit breakers? On the other end are clinical factors and the therapists' skills. Groups provide a unique vehicle for support, feedback, and interpersonal learning. Although daunting, when you manage these many tasks responsibly, you provide a genuine opportunity for the group members to transform with integrity.

GUIDELINES FOR BEGINNING A GROUP

1. Before beginning, talk with your administrators and cofacilitators and discuss the purpose, nature, and function of the group.

2. Set up the physical space for your group with an eye toward safety and adequate comfort.

3. Limit your first group to six members.

4. Choose people for the group who are easy to work with, who you like, and who say they are willing to work with you.

5. Work with a cofacilitator.

6. Run a group in a facility in which you do not work. As was discussed earlier, this prevents burnout and enhances the status of the group being run.

7. Stop to review your work after 12 sessions—identify problem areas, notice the strengths, and determine a direction.

8. Videotape as many of your initial groups as you can.

9. Process your group with your cofacilitator. Watch the videos, talk about what could be done differently, and, most importantly, note what was good about what you did in the group. Serve as teachers and validators for each other.

10. Start a peer support/supervision group to discuss ongoing issues with your groups. Meet a minimum of once a month to review problems and successes that may have come up in running the groups.

11. Get supervision by someone who is experienced in working with the population you are working with and with group process.

12. Attend trainings, read articles, and review training videos that pertain to your group.

APPENDICES

APPENDICES

GLOSSARY

Acceptance. A therapeutic factor. Members feel a sense of belonging and being valued by each other. (Often, members begin looking forward to the group meetings and show up early to set the chairs in a circle. They speak of membership in the group with a sense of pride and importance. There is value placed on being part of the group and, in turn, attendance at the regular meetings creates a feeling of membership.)

Affirmation Stage. The final stage in the Interactive-Behavioral Therapy (IBT) model in which the participants are affirmed by the facilitators and other members for their participation in the group.

Altruism. A therapeutic factor. Members are helpful to others in the group and learn how good it feels. (The emergence of altruism is often one of the first therapeutic factors to occur in the formation of an Interactive-Behavioral Therapy group. The facilitator should be sensitive to any helping gestures and acknowledge them. When one member moves a chair for another, when someone passes a box of tissues to a member because he or she is crying, and when one member volunteers to double for another, are all examples of altruistic behaviors.)

Auxiliary. A role assumed by members in the group other than the protagonist.

Catharsis. A therapeutic factor. A release of an intense feeling that brings about relief for the individual expressing it. While catharsis is often thought of as the purging of a negative emotion, intensely humorous outbursts also can be cathartic.

CGP (Certified Group Psychotherapist). A national certification offered for group psychotherapy.

Closed Group. A group that is not open to new members.

Cohesion. See Acceptance.

Confidentiality. The contract between members that holds them responsible for keeping information shared in the group private.

Contraindication. Signs that a technique or method should not be used.

Corrective Recapitulation of the Primary Family. A therapeutic factor. Members work through feelings established in the family of origin and come to a corrective understanding of those feelings within the group.

Development of Social Skills. A therapeutic factor referring to the feedback available to members from the group concerning social interaction.

Deviant Person. The person in the group most different from the other members.

Double. An action method in which a person's thoughts and feelings, particularly those that may be unexpressed, are spoken by another person. The position of the double, unless contraindicated, is behind the person for whom the double is given. Doubles may be in singles, pairs, or multiples.

Empty Chair. An action method in which a vacant chair is used to symbolize another person or role.

Enactment Stage. The stage when the action takes place in traditional psychodramas and in the IBT model.

Encounter. Any interaction between members, between a protagonist and an auxiliary, between a protagonist and an object (e.g., an empty chair or prop being used in the drama), or between the protagonist and an imaginary figure can be called an encounter. The essence of the "meeting of the two," as Moreno put it, is conflict and the therapeutic struggle for each person or entity to understand each other through empathic awareness. The encounter often is followed by a role reversal.

Existential Factor. A therapeutic factor. The common bonds of inevitable death, loneliness, and suffering are shared by group members.

Fish Bowl. In this training technique, part of the group demonstrates a technique or process while other members of the group observe. This is particularly useful when the group is too large for all members to participate directly.

Gestalt Therapy. Developed in New York in the late 1950s and early 1960s by Frederick (Fritz) and Laura Perls, Paul Goodman, Ralph Hefferline, and others. This form of group therapy became popular when Fritz Perls moved to the Esalen Institute in California around 1966. Perls's version of gestalt therapy is most closely associated with the action methods of psychodrama. Generally speaking, Perls used monodramas in his groups by having a protagonist act out all the parts of a drama him- or herself.

Guidance. A therapeutic factor. Members receive useful information in the form of advice, suggestions, and examples from other members or the facilitator.

Heterogeneous. In group therapy, refers to differences among members.

Homogeneous. In group therapy, refers to similarities among members.

Horizontal Self-Disclosure. See Self-Disclosure.

IBT. Interactive-Behavioral Therapy. (See pages 147–156 and Chapter 9.)

Imparting of Information (Education). A therapeutic factor. The didactic element in the group—providing information for the purpose of education.

Instillation of Hope. A therapeutic factor. Members gain optimism from being in the group and from witnessing change in others.

Intrapsychic Conflict. An internal conflict within an individual's psyche.

Isomorphic. A condition where the external stimuli match or resonate with the internal stimuli.

Interpersonal Action. A therapeutic factor. Learning that happens as a by-product of relating to other people. (The format of the group allows for a relatively high degree of structure within which the group norms are set and members can learn through interaction how best to accommodate to the norms.)

Modeling. A therapeutic factor. Exhibiting a desirable behavior such that others learn by witnessing and imitating it.

Monodrama. A drama in which the protagonist plays all the parts him- or herself. As such this type of drama is done without the use of auxiliaries.

Multiple Double. When a number of people double for a protagonist.

Observing Ego. The part of our awareness that can view our behaviors, thoughts, feelings, or reactions with sufficient detachment to provide new perspectives or understandings.

Open Group. A group in which new members join as others leave.

Orientation Stage. The first stage in the IBT model. Members interact with one another through participation.

OTR. Outpatient Treatment Report. (See pages 30–31.)

Paired Double. When two doubles take opposite perspectives to heighten a conflict or introduce alternate ways of thinking and feeling.

Polarity. One end of a spectrum of possibilities.

Projection. In psychodrama, the distortions of the protagonist that are vented onto an empty chair or auxiliaries.

Protagonist. The central figure in a drama. In action methods, the individual who acts out his or her scene for the group.

Psychoeducational Group. A group that deals with psychological problems by imparting of information (education). For example, a psychoeducational group might give family members information on the effects of alcoholism on the body and the impact the alcoholic has on the family.

Reciprocal Choice. This refers to the fact that two members of the group are choosing each other and a mutual attraction is present.

Role Prescription. The protagonist, usually through role reversal, provides auxiliaries with the specific dynamics of a role.

Role Reversal. Alternating roles during a drama. The actors physically reverse their positions and take on the character of the other person.

Scene Setting. Establishing an environment in the group setting that will create a scene.

Self-Disclosure. A therapeutic factor. Personal information given by one person to other(s). Horizontal self-disclosure refers to less emotionally charged information. Vertical self-disclosure pertains to more in-depth feelings.

Self-Understanding. A therapeutic factor. Members learn something important about themselves through feedback from others in the group.

Sharing Stage. The stage at the end of the group where members discuss their insights and observations. (Not to be confused with advice giving.)

Social Skills Development. See Development of Social Skills.

Sociodynamic Energy. Term given to measure the degree to which we are drawn to, repulsed by, or are neutral to others. Both the intensity and the direction of this energy can vary from person to person and condition to condition.

Sociometry. A measure of the strength of attraction between and among people based on different criteria.

Spectrogram. A sociometric technique designed to measure the range of responses to a question. People stand along a continuum of two polarities to identify their status. (This technique is used to help people begin interacting with one another while noting their relationship to others in the group.)

Tele. The natural interconnections that exist between and among people; often referred to as "chemistry" or "vibes."

Therapeutic Factors. Factors thought to be of benefit to people in psychotherapeutic treatment. (The term was made popular in the field by Irving Yalom.)

Transference. Feelings previously experienced toward one person transferred to another.

Training Group. A group designed for the purpose of training group psychotherapists. Such a group involves aspects of actual group therapy along with didactic presentations and reading material.

Universality. A therapeutic factor. The discovery that one's issues, problems, perceptions, and concerns are not unique. (Once members know that others can relate to them, there is relief in the kinship.)

Vertical Self-Disclosure. See Self-Disclosure.

Vicarious Learning. See Modeling.

Warm-Up and Sharing Stage. The second stage in the Interactive-Behavioral Therapy model when participants describe what issues they would like to work on.

Warm-Up Stage. The stage at the beginning of the group when members ready themselves for the work or action or task of the group.

RESOURCES

SEMINAL WORKS OF J. L. MORENO

Jacob L. Moreno, M.D. (1889-1974) is the founder of psychodrama and sociometry and a pioneer in group psychotherapy. His major works are now out of print but may be available through companies such as amazon.com. Also, many university libraries may have copies of or access to his work. See the References for a listing of titles.

BOOKS ON PSYCHODRAMA, SOCIOMETRY, AND PSYCHOTHERAPY

Bernard, H., & MacKenzie, K. (Eds). (1994). *Basics of group psychotherapy*. New York: Guilford.

Blatner, A. (1996). *Acting in*. New York: Springer.

Blatner, A. (1987). *Foundations of psychodrama: History, theory and practice*. New York: Springer.

Frost, J. H., & Wilmot, W. (1978). *Interpersonal conflict* (pp. 144-147). Dubuque, IA: Wm. C. Brown.

Fuhlrodt, R. B. (Ed.). (1990). *Psychodrama: Its application to ACOA and substance abuse treatment.* (Available from Perrin & Teggett Booksellers, P.O. Box 190, Rutherford, NJ 07070.

Gazda, G. M. (Ed.). (1982). *Basic approaches to group psychotherapy and group counseling* (3rd ed.). Springfield, IL: Charles C. Thomas.

Greenberg, I. A. (Ed.). (1974). *Psychodrama: Theory and therapy.* New York: Behavioral Publications.

Hale, A. E. (1986). *Conducting clinical sociometric explorations: A manual for psychodramatists and sociometrists.* (Available from Anne E. Hale, 1601 Memorial Avenue #4, Roanoke, VA 24015).

Hollander, C. E. (1978). *A process for psychodrama training: The Hollander psychodrama curve.* Denver, CO: Snow Lion Press.

Holmes, P. H. (1992). *The inner world outside: Object relations and psychodrama.* London: Tavistock/Routledge.

Hornyak, L. M., & Baker, E. K. (Eds.). (1989). *Experimental therapies for eating disorders.* New York: Guilford.

Hudgins, M. K., & Kiesler, D. J. (1984). *Instructional manual for doubling in individual psychotherapy.* (Available from The Center for Experiential Learning, 3440 Lake Mendota Drive, Madison, WI 53705).

Kipper, D. A. (1986). *Psychotherapy through clinical role-playing.* New York: Brunner/Mazel.

Kumar, V. K., & Treadwell, T. W. (1985). *Practical sociometry for psychodramatist.* (Available from Tom W. Treadwell, West Chester University, West Chester, PA 19380).

ADDITIONAL RESOURCES

The following resources are provided to help practitioners continue with their professional growth.

- For information on becoming a Certified Group Psychotherapist, contact the National Registry of Certified Group Psychotherapists, 25 East 21st Street, 6th Floor, New York, NY 10010. Phone 212-477-1600, Fax 212-979-6627.

- For a review copy and information on the training video and manual *Interactive-Behavioral on Group Counseling for People with Mild and Moderate Mental Retardation*, please contact Young Adult Institute, 460 West 34th Street, New York, NY 10001. Phone 212-563-7474, Fax 212- 268-1083.

- For an extensive, continuously updated bibliography on psychodrama, sociodrama, and related techniques and theory, contact James M. Sacks, Ph.D. T.E.P., Psychodrama Center of New York, 71 Washington Place, New York, NY 10011-9184.

- For information on training facilities as well as publication opportunities and certification in group psychotherapy and psychodrama, contact The American Society for Group Psychotherapy and Psychodrama (ASGPP), 301 North Harrison Street, Suite 508, Princeton, NJ 08540. Phone 609-452-1339, Fax 609-452-1659. Website: http://artswire.org/asgpp/index.html.

- For copies of the *International Journal of Action Methods, Psychodrama, Skill Training, and Role Playing,* contact Heldref Publications, 1319 Eighteenth Street, NW, Washington, DC 20036-1802. Phone 1-800-365-9753.

- For current information on group therapy from Division 49 of the American Psychological Association, contact APA at 1-800-374-2721 and ask for the current mailing address and phone numbers.

- For on-site training, conferences, and inquiries about training in group psychotherapy, contact Daniel J. Tomasulo, Ph.D., T.E.P., CGP, 723 North Beers Street, Suite # 2B, Holmdel, NJ 07733. Phone 732-264-9501, Fax 732-264-8135, e-mail tomasulo@worldnet.att.net.

REFERENCES

Blatner, A. (1985). The dynamics of cartharsis. *Journal of Group Psychotherapy, Psychodrama and Sociometry, 37*(4), 157–166.

Blatner, A. (1996). *Acting–in. Second edition.* New York: Springer.

Blatner A, & Blatner, A. (1988). *Foundations of psychodrama history: Theory and practice.* New York: Springer.

Bloch S, & Crouch, E. (1985). *Therapeutic factors in group psychotherapy.* New York: Oxford University Press.

Buchanan, D. R. (1984). Program analysis of a centralized psychotherapy service in a large mental hospital. *Journal of Group Psychotherapy, Psychodrama and Sociometry, 37*, 32–40.

Buchanan, D. R., & Dubbs-Siroka, J. (1980). Psychodramatic treatment for psychiatric patients. *Journal of the National Association of Private Psychiatric Hospitals, 11*, 27–31.

Cox, M., Taplin, O., Berry, C., Roine, E., Meyer, M. A., Hewish, S., & Saunders, J. (1992). Drama in custodial settings. In M. Cox (Ed.), *Shakespeare comes to Broadmoor: "The actors are come hither": The performance of tragedy in a secure psychiatric hospital.* London: Jessica Kingsley.

223

Fletcher R. (1984). Group therapy with mentally retarded persons with emotional disorders. *Psychiatric Aspects of Mental Retardation Reviews, 3,* 21–24.

Fox, J. (Ed.). (1987). *The essential Moreno: Writings on psychodrama group method and spontaneity by J. L. Moreno, M.D.* New York: Springer.

Hingsburger, D. (1987). Sex counseling with the developmentally handicapped: The assessment and management of seven critical problems. *Psychiatric Aspects of Mental Retardation Reviews, 6,* 41–46.

Hurley, A. D. (1989). Individual psychotherapy with mentally retarded individuals: A review and call for research. *Research in Developmental Disabilities, 10,* 261–275.

Hurley, A. D., & Hurley, F. J.(1986) Counseling and psychotherapy with mentally retarded clients: I. The initial interview. *Psychiatric Aspects of Mental Retardation Reviews, 5,* 22–26.

Hurley, A. D., & Hurley, F. J. (1988). Counseling and psychotherapy with mentally retarded clients: II. Establishing a relationship. *Psychiatric Aspects of Mental Retardation Reviews, 6,* 15–20,.

Hurley, A., Pfadt, A., Tomasulo, D., & Gardner, W. (1996). Counseling and psychotherapy. In J. Jacobson & J. Mulick (Eds.), *Manual of diagnosis and professional practice in mental retardation.* Washington, DC: American Psychological Association.

Keller, E. (1995). Process and outcomes in Interactive-Behavioral Groups with adults who have both mental illness and mental retardation. Unpublished doctoral dissertation, Long Island University, C.W. Post Campus.

Marineau, R. (1990). *Jacob Levy Moreno, 1889-1974.* London: Tavistock/ Routledge.

Matson, J. L. (1985). Biosocial theory of psychopathology: A three factor model. *Applied Research in Mental Retardation, 6,* 199–227.

Moreno, J. L. (1946). *Psychodrama* (Vol. 1). Beacon, NY: Beacon House.

Moreno, J. L. (1947). *Theatre of spontaneity: An introduction to psychodrama.* Beacon, NY: Beacon House.

Moreno, J. L. (1951). *Sociometry: Experimental method and the science of sociometry.* Beacon, NY: Beacon House.

Moreno, J. L. (Ed.). (1956). *Sociometry and the science of man.* Beacon, NY: Beacon House.

Moreno, J. L. (1978). *Who shall survive?* (3rd ed.). Beacon, NY: Beacon House.

Moreno, J. L., & Moreno, Z. T. (1959). *Psychodrama* (Vol. 2). Beacon, NY: Beacon House.

Pfadt A. (1991). Group psychotherapy with mentally retarded adults: Issues related to design, implementation and evaluation. *Res Dev Disabil, 12,* 261–285.

Pirsig, R. (1974). *Zen and the art of motorcycle maintenance.* New York: Morrow.

Poeys. (1985). Guidelines for the practice of brief, dynamic group therapy. *International Journal of Group Psychotherapy, 35,* 331–354.

Razza, N., & Tomasulo, D. (1996a). The sexual abuse continuum: Therapeutic interventions with individuals with mental retardation. *Habil Mental Healthcare Newsletter, 15,* 19–22.

Razza, N., & Tomasulo, D. (1996b). The sexual abuse continuum: Part 2. Therapeutic interventions with individuals with mental retardation. *Habil Mental Healthcare Newsletter, 15,* 84–86.

Razza, N., & Tomasulo, D. (1996c). The sexual abuse continuum: Part 3. Therapeutic interventions with individuals with mental retardation. *Habil Mental Healthcare Newsletter, 15,* 116–119.

Schramski, T. (1984). Role-playing as a therapeutic approach with the mentally retarded. *Psychiatric Aspects of Mental Retardation Reviews, 3,* 26–32.

Siroka, R. W., & Schloss, G. A. (1968). The death scene in psychodrama. *Group Psychotherapy, 21,* 202–205. [Reprinted (1968). *Psychopharmaceutica and Techniques in Group Psychotherapy,* 355–361.]

Spencer, P. G., Gillespie, C. R., & Ekisa, E. G. (1983). A controlled comparison of the effects of social skills training and remedial drama on the conversational skills of chronic schizophrenic inpatients. *British Journal of Psychiatry, 143,* 165–172.

Starr, A., & Weisz, H. S. (1989). Psychodramatic techniques in the brief treatment of inpatient groups. *Individual Psychology: Journal of Adlerian Theory, Research and Practice, 45,* 143–147.

Steinberg, P., & Garcia, A. (1989). *Sociodrama: Who's in your shoes?* New York: Praeger.

Tomasulo, D. (1990). *Interactive-behavioral group counseling for people with mild and moderate retardation* [video]. (Available from Young Adult Institute, 460 West 34th Street, New York, NY 10001.)

Tomasulo D. (1992). *Interactive–behavioral group counseling for people with mild to moderate mental retardation* (two videos). New York: Young Adult Institute.

Tomasulo, D. (1994). Action techniques in group counseling: The double. *Habil Mental Healthcare Newsletter, 13,* 41–45.

Tomasulo, D. (1997). Beginning and maintaining a group. *Habil Mental Healthcare Newsletter, 16*(3), 41–48.

Tomasulo, D. (1998). Substance abuse: Who will do it? *Mental Health Aspects of Developmental Disabilities, 1,* 20–22.

Tomasulo, D, Keller, E, & Pfadt, A. (1995). The healing crowd. *Habil Mental Healthcare Newsletter, 14,* 43–50.

Woods, & Melnick. (1979). A review of group therapy selection criteria. *Small Group Behavior, 10,* 155–175.

Yalom, I. (1983). *Inpatient group psychotherapy.* New York: Basic Books.

Yalom, I. (1995). *Group psychotherapy* (4th ed.). New York: Basic Books.

Index

ABOUT THE AUTHOR

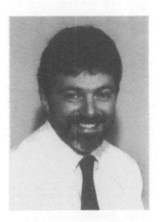

Photo by Joel Morgovsky

Daniel J. Tomasulo, Ph.D., T.E.P., CGP, is a psychologist, trainer, educator, practitioner of psychodrama, and certified group psychotherapist who has gained national recognition for his development of the Interactive-Behavioral Therapy (IBT) model of group psychotherapy for people with mental retardation and chronic psychiatric disabilities. He is Professor of Psychology at Brookdale

College and a psychological consultant for the Young Adult Institute. He also has served on fellowship at Princeton University as visiting faculty. Dr. Tomasulo is the author of numerous professional publications and is a fellow of the American Society for Group Psychotherapy and Psychodrama. He is past president of the New Jersey chapter and the recipient of the ASGPP's Innovator's Award for his development of the IBT model of group psychotherapy.

T - #0527 - 101024 - C0 - 229/152/13 - PB - 9781560326595 - Gloss Lamination